TONE every INCH.™

TONE
every
INCH™

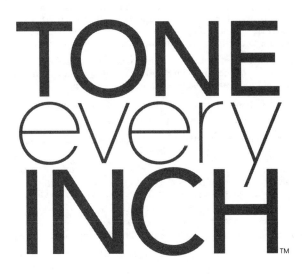

THE FASTEST WAY TO SCULPT YOUR BELLY, BUTT & THIGHS

Natalie Gingerich Mackenzie
with the editors of **Prevention**®

RODALE®

© 2012 by Rodale Inc.

Exclusive direct hardcover and trade paperback published simultaneously by Rodale Inc. in January 2012.

Rodale books may be purchased for business or promotional use or for special sales. For information, please write to:
Special Markets Department, Rodale Inc., 733 Third Avenue, New York, NY 10017

Prevention and Tone Every Inch are registered trademarks of Rodale Inc.

Printed in the United States of America

Rodale Inc. makes every effort to use acid-free ♾, recycled paper ♻.

Exercise photographs by Mitch Mandel/Rodale Inc.

Profile photographs by Jon Reis Photography

Book design by Carol Angstadt

Library of Congress Cataloging-in-Publication Data
Mackenzie, Natalie Gingerich.
    Tone every inch: The fastest way to sculpt your belly, butt & thighs / Natalie Gingerich Mackenzie with the editors of Prevention.
        p.   cm.
    Includes index.
    ISBN 978-1-60961-243-6   direct hardcover
    ISBN 978-1-60961-742-4   trade paperback
    1. Physical fitness.   2. Weight training.   3. Bodybuilding.   I. Title.
RA781.M3167   2012
613.7—dc23   2011036585

Distributed to the trade by Macmillan

            2   4   6   8   10   9   7   5   3   1   direct hardcover

            2   4   6   8   10   9   7   5   3   1   trade paperback

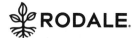

We inspire and enable people to improve their lives and the world around them.
For more of our products visit **prevention.com**

To all the strong women

I've had the opportunity to meet,

write about, and

be inspired by in my life:

This book is for you.

Contents

Introduction

The seeds for this book were planted back in 2008, before I left my job as fitness editor at *Prevention* magazine to become a full-time freelance writer. The magazine's then-editorial assistant Danielle Kosecki stumbled upon a groundbreaking study revealing that something as simple as pairing a dumbbell with a stretchy elastic resistance band could not merely double—but triple—your toning results. We couldn't wait to share this incredible finding with our readers, and we immediately enlisted Danielle to write about it for our October 2008 issue. The initial article was a short item in *Prevention*'s News and Trends section with three exercises to try using the method. But we weren't done. Eight months later, in the June 2009 issue, we featured a second combo band-and-dumbbell routine, this time expanding it to eight head-to-toe moves.

But I couldn't help being bothered by the fact that this training style we were all so excited about was based on research on college kids—and athletes at that. Many exercise studies are done at universities worldwide because students are the easiest subjects to come by (not to mention the easiest to bribe with bonuses like extra-credit points and raffles for free pizza). Not that I doubted the efficacy of the program. In fact, one study I had read by a team of Brazilian researchers who presented their work at the American College of Sports Medicine annual conference actually compared the results of a group of 18- to 35-year-old women and a group of women over age 60 who embarked on the same twice-a-week strength and cardio routine. Contrary to those who say you have to go slow when you get older, this study found that not only were the older women no more likely to get injured, but they also gained strength at exactly the same rate as the younger ones. Better still, they improved their aerobic endurance by 20 percent more than the mostly 20-somethings. But I wanted to see it for myself.

So I enlisted the help of an exercise science research class at Ithaca College in New York. We put together a study plan, got our methods approved by the college's Human Subjects Research board, and advertised everywhere from the public library to Craigslist.org. Our target: women over age 35 with jobs, kids, and carpools who wanted to finally get in shape. The women we found weren't all couch potatoes. Several of them walked their dogs daily; others liked to hike, do Pilates, or even lift weights occasionally. And yes, some hadn't exercised in years. But what they all had in common was the frustration that what they were doing wasn't working, and they were ready to try something new. Enter: *Tone Every Inch.*

Our team of a dozen women got a preview of the plan in this book nearly a year before it was printed. After being weighed and measured, they did the exercises for 8 weeks, coming in after Week 3 (the end of Phase 2) and Week 8 to see how they'd progressed. The results didn't disappoint. Even Barbara Terrell, who already lifted weights regularly at the start of the program, gained an astounding 25 percent more strength in her upper body (measured by how much she could bench-press five times) and 32 percent more strength in her lower body (measured by how much she could lift five times on a leg press machine). Test panelists took off as many as 11 pounds during the initial program and continued to lose even after the 8 weeks. They headed into summer feeling confident in shorts and swimsuits, and they impressed their kids who came home from college to fitter-than-ever moms. The only complaints I heard as we were wrapping up the study: "I wish I'd done this sooner" and "I'd forgotten how amazing it feels" to be in good shape.

Now it's your turn to reap the benefits and tone every inch! I'm eager to share with you this amazingly simple yet effective program to help you lose weight, trim inches, and firm up in just 30 minutes a day. Let's get started!

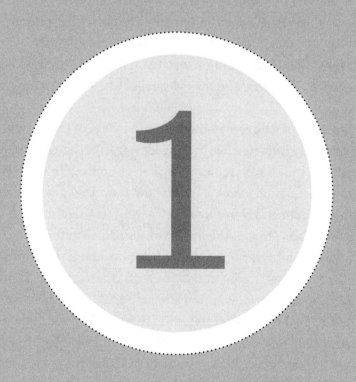

Why Muscle Matters

I love exercise. Without it, I get cranky and hard to be around, as my husband will be the first to tell you. In fact, I love it so much that I've made it my career, writing about fitness for magazines including *Prevention*. But I'm going to let you in on a little secret:

1

I didn't always love strength training. Like roughly 25 million other Americans, I like to run. I also love walking and hiking with my dog, Charley. Strength training was always something I thought of as extra credit I meant to do when things got a little less crazy and I was able to find the time (but really, who has extra time?). And did I mention I'm not a huge fan of gyms? But let me tell you something. After years of interviewing trainers and PhDs and reading study after study about the many benefits of strength training, it's hard not to be convinced.

Age and the Slow Calorie Creep

After all, it turns out that even if you walk or run regularly like I do, if you take a hands-off approach to dumbbells, you start losing ½ pound of muscle a year as early as your twenties. Think losing ½ pound a year of anything doesn't seem like much to worry about? Think again. Because muscle burns more calories than fat does, it's what keeps your metabolism humming along at an I-can-have-a-cookie-and-not-feel-guilty rate.

Here's how Wayne Westcott, PhD, who led exercise studies on thousands of ordinary folks as the fitness research director at South Shore YMCA in Quincy, Massachusetts, explains it: Add those yearly half pounds up over a decade and that measly fraction of a pound a year means a difference of up to 5 percent in your basal metabolic rate (BMR), the calories you burn even if you stay in bed all day. For the sake of simple math, let's say your do-nothing metabolism is 1,200 calories a day. (It's probably a bit higher—you can estimate yours by plugging your info into the formula in "Do the Math: How to Calculate Your Basal Metabolic Rate.") Five percent of those 1,200 daily calories is just 60 calories—not much, right? Maybe not in just 1 day, but let's do some math.

First of all, because the increase to an extra 60 calories a day is happening over the course of a decade, let's average it out to 30 extra calories a day (the number will be lower in the first 5 years and higher in the last 5). Given that it takes 3,500 extra calories to make a pound of fat, those 30 little calories multiplied by 365 days a year equal a little more than 3 pounds each year. Over 10 years, 30 calories a day adds up to a noticeable 30 pounds.

DO THE MATH: HOW TO CALCULATE YOUR BASAL METABOLIC RATE

Want to know approximately how many calories you burn each day without exercising? Plug your height, weight, and age into the formula below, and then punch it all into a calculator to get your number.

$$655 + (4.35 \times \textbf{weight in pounds}) + (4.7 \times \textbf{height in inches})$$
$$- (4.7 \times \textbf{age in years}) = \textbf{BMR}$$

Now what? Remember, your BMR is an estimate of your baseline calorie burn. Everything you do from standing up and reaching for a book on the top shelf to working out on the treadmill adds to that number. To estimate your actual calorie burn, there's something called the Harris Benedict Equation, which gives you a number to multiply your BMR by depending on how active you are.

If you get little or no exercise: Multiply by 1.2.

If you exercise lightly one to three times per week: Multiply by 1.375.

If you exercise moderately three to five times per week: Multiply by 1.55.

If you exercise hard six or seven times per week: Multiply by 1.725.

If you exercise very hard and have a physical job: Multiply by 1.9.

Even the Skinny Aren't Safe

Now, if you look at a picture of yourself in college compared to the you who shows up in the mirror these days and that gradual weight gain sounds about right, you might be sold. But here's the kicker: Even if you *haven't gained a pound* since your early twenties, if you're not strength training, this is still happening to you. Even if you haven't become overweight, there's a good chance you are what's called overfat.

In fact, a study from the Mayo Clinic in Rochester, Minnesota, looked at this exact phenomenon. The researchers measured the body fat percentage of more than 1,000 women (average age 41) whose weight appeared healthy on the scale. Guess what: 54 percent of them clocked in at more than 30 percent body fat, earning them the designation of "normal weight obese" (18.5 to 24.9 percent is considered a healthy body fat for women, 25 to 29.9 percent is considered overweight, and 30 percent or higher is considered obese, according to the researchers).

Turns out this normal weight obesity (otherwise known as being skinny fat) means more than being a little soft underneath single digit–size clothing. The researchers found that women with a body fat percentage greater than 30 percent—even with a seemingly healthy weight and BMI—had nearly four times the chance of also being diagnosed with metabolic syndrome. That's a cluster of risk factors (including insulin resistance, high cholesterol, and extra weight around the midsection) that increases your propensity for heart disease, stroke, and type 2 diabetes; doubles your risk of high triglycerides; triples the risk of prediabetes; and leads to a 20 percent jump in high blood pressure compared to women with less body fat.

How to Beat Calorie Creep

The best way to beat those odds? Exercise. And an essential ingredient of that exercise is strength training, which gives your body composition a one-two punch by simultaneously reducing fat while increasing muscle. (Your body composition is the balance of fat and lean tissue in your body.) Try to lose weight with diet alone and you're liable to lose more muscle, worsening your body's fat-to-lean ratio.

Take a 150-pound woman with a body fat percentage of 33 percent. That means her body is made up of about 50 pounds of fat, and 100 pounds of muscle, bone, and connective tissue—basically everything else that's not fat. If she loses 10 pounds of fat, she's now 140 pounds, and she's lowered her body fat percentage to 28 percent (40 remaining pounds of fat divided by the 140 pounds she now weighs). But the picture is different if she loses the same 10 pounds but they come from muscle. Now she's reduced her weight to 140 pounds, but she still has 50 pounds of fat on her frame. Divide those numbers and now she's almost 36 percent fat—an increase in her body fat percentage as a result of *losing* weight.

In real life, that's an extreme example. Cutting calories is most likely to yield weight loss that's a combination of fat and muscle loss. When researchers at the University of Westminster, London, dug through 147 studies comparing different diets, exercise routines, and combinations of diets and exercise routines, they found evidence that even the most effective diets could easily shave off as much metabolism-fueling muscle as they did fat—if they didn't incorporate exercise.

In fact, in one University of Cincinnati study reviewed by the London researchers, dieters on a low-carb plan lost 6.7 percent body fat (good) as well as 6.8 percent lean body weight (not good!). The net impact is that they finished the diet slimmer, but burning 82 fewer calories a day. Talk about a recipe for regain! For lasting weight loss and an improved body composition ratio, researchers found that the most effective plan for both losing weight and preserving lean muscle mass is strength training and high-intensity cardio combined with a healthy diet rich in protein and fiber—the very stuff this program is built on.

Face-Off: Dumbbells vs. Dieting

So far we've talked about how *not* strength training can trigger the slow creep of weight over the years. But what's done is done, you say. What is lifting weights going to do to help me take it off? I'm glad you asked! You probably know that there are a few different things you can do to lose weight (and maybe you've tried them all more times than you can count).

You could diet, right? In fact, some might say that dieting is the easiest way to take off weight, and they'd probably be right. After all, other than the willpower required to pass on an extra scoop of ice cream, it doesn't actually take much time or physical effort to *not* eat. But there's a dark side to dieting by cutting calories only—it leaves you vulnerable to weight regain. Worse still, you're actually likely to gain back everything you lost *and then some.* Talk about a buzz kill—all that willpower for nothing!

In a perfect world, passing on greasy fast food or a rich, creamy hunk of cheesecake would translate into the loss of similarly fatty stuff on our bodies. But scientists haven't found that to be true. Actually, when you're losing weight, your body likes to hang on to its fat stores, which turn out to be a good rainy day energy store (you know, in case there's a famine), and instead use stores of lean muscle tissue. By losing weight this way, you're actually slowing down your metabolism.

That means when you finally relax from your diet, the same number of calories you used to eat to maintain your old weight will now be enough to spur weight gain. Take the University of Cincinnati study we talked about before. After losing weight (and a significant amount of muscle), if the subjects were to go forth eating the same number of calories they'd needed to maintain their weights before, they'd gain almost 9 pounds in the coming year. If you've yo-yoed from diet to diet for years, hopefully this helps to elucidate why the results never seem to stick.

Fighting Fat with Muscle

But there's a better way. By adding exercise—specifically strength training—into the mix, you'll prevent some of the muscle loss associated with both age and diet-focused weight loss. And even better (here's the good part), you'll add new muscle to kick-start your calorie burn as well as train the muscle to be a better fat burner. In fact, based on several well-regarded studies on the subject, researchers have concluded that a typical strength-training program can boost your burn by about 7 percent, or about 100 calories a day. Make no other changes and that's good for a loss of about 10 pounds a year. Not bad, huh?

Plus, muscle is denser than fat, so pound for pound it takes up about 18 percent less space (read: helps you to shed inches as well as pounds), is firmer (goodbye, jiggly upper arms!), and may be one of the best tools in your arsenal against cellulite because it helps to firm flesh that might otherwise be susceptible to puckering, according to a study by Dr. Westcott.

But we're not clueless. Given the current statistics in the United States, 68 percent of us are overweight, while half again of that number qualify as obese. So while 10 pounds is a great start, many of you are probably looking to lose more than that, and many others simply want to do it in less than a year. If you're ready for the challenge, this program is, too. First of all, the 100 calories a day mentioned above refer only to the increase in your baseline metabolism—the number we talked about above. We haven't even given you credit for the calories you'll burn exercising! Let's start with strength training.

Oh, the Calories You'll Burn

At face value, strength training may not seem like much of a fat blaster (hence the reason so many Americans who are trying to lose weight head for the treadmill instead of the dumbbells). It's true, a typical 30-minute strength-training session burns between 100 and 200 calories depending on how hard you work. Trade that for fast walking or jogging and you could practically double that number in the same amount of time. So why not spend your precious time on cardio?

Well, besides the benefits of strong muscles we already talked about, the calories you burn during strength training are only part of the story. Challenging your muscles creates a metabolic spike that lasts even after you shower and change your clothes—as long as 12 hours, according to some studies. Moreover, research has shown that during a bout of strength training, the body's fat-burning engines are cranked up to 78 percent, and that extra burn continues for 40 minutes afterward. The total day's haul: twice the fat burn compared with not exercising.

BREAKING THE STRENGTH STIGMA: YOU WON'T BULK UP

Between you and me, I haven't met too many women who want to bulk up, period. And that fear is one of the reasons too many women bypass strength training. It's true that when you train your muscles, one of the adaptations that occurs within the muscle fibers is that they grow larger, a phenomenon called hypertrophy. In addition to fueling 24/7 calorie burn, this is what helps firm your skin, reducing the look of cellulite and flabbiness, as well as giving your arms, legs, and butt a nice sculpted shape. Nobody wants a flat derriere, but with the loss of muscle mass as you head into middle age, that seems to be one of the first shape changes to take place in men and women of all sizes. What I'm saying is, you may not want to "bulk up," but you *do* want the benefits of increasing the size of those muscle fibers.

That said, it's true that some of us are more prone to a muscular build than others. I know because I'm one of those people. In fact, I have been asked by strangers how I got such muscular legs—and that's when I wasn't doing any sort of strength training at all. In my case, I chalk it up to

Your Recipe for Success

Despite all these great benefits of strength training, I'm not suggesting that you should skip cardio altogether, or that dieting is doomed. In fact, I'll explain more in the coming chapters, but the program in this book relies on a combination of muscle strengthening, cardio, and healthy eating. It's depressing but true that only about 1 in 6 dieters successfully keeps the weight off for the long term, in part because of some of the factors we discussed above.

So for a more optimistic view, let's take a look at what did work for those who have been successful at changing their bodies for the long run. The National Weight Control Registry, a collaboration that began in 1994 between researchers from Brown Medical School and the University of Colorado, has grown to become the largest ongoing investigation into running (how's that for a "high rep" exercise!) but mostly genetics. And I (try to) embrace my musculature for the ability it gives me to run fast, eat ice cream, and carry on a tradition of women in my family with shapely, powerful legs. After all, firm beats flabby any day of the week! Strength training, on the other hand, has never made my already less-than-spindly legs any bigger. In fact, while I've never whipped out a measuring tape, I'd venture that training with weights and bands makes them leaner by helping to shrink fat cells and tighten and tone the muscle I already have.

But that's anecdotal. Let's check out the results of our test panel to see how they did in the bulking-up department. On average, the women on our panel increased their upper-body strength by 14 percent by the end of the program, yet the size of their upper arms decreased by an average of $\frac{2}{10}$ inch. In fact, the two women who gained the most upper-body strength—20 and 25 percent, respectively—also shrunk their upper arms by nearly $\frac{1}{2}$ inch and a full inch. In the lower body, our testers boosted their strength by an average of 21 percent while subtracting an average of $1\frac{1}{2}$ inches from their hips and thighs.

what works in losing weight and keeping it off. The researchers maintain a database of more than 5,000 members who have lost an average of 66 pounds and kept it off for 5 or more years. And guess what: 90 percent of them rely on a combination of exercise and healthy eating to stay slim.

In another study looking at about 100 women who had previously lost an average of 24 pounds, researchers followed up with the women for a year, keeping tabs on whether they continued to do strength or aerobic exercise. The result: Those who completely stopped exercising gained back 33 percent of the dangerous visceral fat around their waistlines. Meanwhile, those who did even 80 minutes a week of strength and cardio gained back none of the dangerous belly fat—none, zero, zilch. Not bad!

But not all exercise plans are created equal, so let's get on with it already and introduce you to this one!

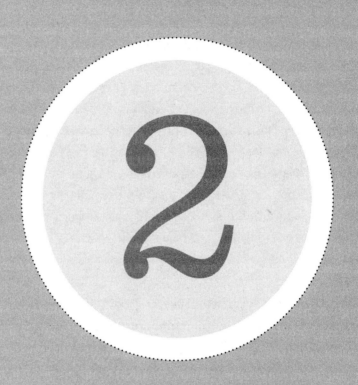

How to Tone Every Inch

If you're with me so far, I hope you're convinced to try this thing called strength training. But the burning question that remains is, what's so special about *this* plan and what sets it apart from all the others out there? I won't lie to you—doing just about any resistance exercise program is better than doing none. But if you're like most women, you have a jam-packed schedule. Finding time to do any sort of exercise can be a challenge, and the last thing you want is to use your precious time any less efficiently than you could.

I've spent the last 8 years writing about fitness for national magazines, reading studies of different exercise programs, and interviewing the PhDs who conduct those studies. If one thing is constant in research on exercise, it's that exercise never really changes but the research never stands still. I often get the question of how I manage to come up with new story ideas month after month, and I'll be the first to admit that it can often feel like slicing and dicing the same potato a million different ways. Many of the most effective moves out there (including the squats and lunges you'll see in this plan) are anything but new or revolutionary. They just work. But researchers keep exploring exactly how they work and how to make them better.

A Truly Revolutionary Approach

But one day I came across a particular research study that really got me excited. Having read my share of studies that nitpicked every possible aspect of exercise, from the lineup of moves to the order in which they're done, this one caught my eye because it was a truly revolutionary approach—and one I'd never seen or thought of before. The researchers took elastic resistance tubing (like the stretchy resistance bands you may have seen before) and combined it with traditional weights. The results? The exercisers who used this combo method of training gained not twice but *three times the strength in just 7 weeks*, compared with peers who did standard-issue dumbbell exercises.

Not bad, you might say, but weren't the doubled-up exercisers lifting twice as much weight? If so, of course they got stronger. Well, I'm glad you asked, because to me that's the most impressive part of this study and the results the researchers found: The resistance was matched so that everybody lifted the same amount (relative to their own strength, that is). And the experimental group *still* gained three whole times the metabolism-fueling, fat-melting, energy-boosting strength as their counterparts lifting boring old dumbbells. Now I don't know about you, but given the option, I'd rather spend my precious exercise minutes on a workout that's been proven to yield triple the benefit, even if it does require picking up an extra piece of equipment!

As fate would have it, a couple of years later my husband's job moved our family just over an hour away from Ithaca, New York, where that original research had been conducted, and when I decided to write this book about strength training, I knew that a follow-up study was in order. Whereas the original research had been done in a gym full of heavy-duty equipment, and the subjects had been college athletes, I didn't see any reason that the very same thing couldn't be done using simple, inexpensive equipment right in your own living room. Moreover, if it worked for already pretty fit 20-somethings, the results should be the same or even better for women over 40.

With fate in my corner again, it just so happened that a fellow alum of my college track team, Miranda Kaye, PhD, was now an assistant professor of exercise science at Ithaca College and was teaching a research methods class. In other words, her students were on the hunt for cool new research to execute, and she thought my proposal of a "real women" redo of the band-plus-dumbbell study sounded like a great idea. Together we approached her colleague Gary Sforzo, PhD, the exercise physiologist and professor of exercise science at Ithaca College who had overseen the original study. He agreed to help us hash out the study design. Add a team of six standout exercise science students to help collect measurements and we were in business.

The Tone Every Inch Program

Obviously this plan is built around the combo training technique described above, but we're not just a one-trick pony. To give you a program that's safe, effective, and well rounded enough to stick with for the long haul, we've put the combo strength-training scheme together with cardio workouts designed to get you in and out in minimum time and with maximum results. Plus, we've paired these workouts with a smart eating plan that will help you lose weight without undercutting the energy you need to complete these workouts and the fuel you need to build metabolism-fueling muscle. Here are a few more of the principles this program is founded on.

The Power of Progression

If you already lift weights but simply haven't seen the results you're looking for, ask yourself a question: When was the last time you changed the dumbbell in your hand? In my admittedly unscientific poll of women who do work out with weights, I'd wager that the number one mistake they make that keeps them from seeing the kind of results I've been talking about is doing the same thing again and again.

You see, exercise is a little like addiction (but in a good way!). When you're starting out, it might take a small amount of resistance to challenge your muscles in a way that stimulates them to get stronger. But if you keep using that same small amount of resistance week after week, month after month, you'll stop seeing the gains you did in the beginning. It's similar to how, for me, a cup-a-day coffee habit has grown to more like three (or occasionally five) as caffeine has become my new "normal." Exercise works the same way. Now that you're fitter than when you began, you need a greater challenge to avoid those dreaded plateaus.

Exercise scientists call it progressive overload, which basically just means that you should turn it up a notch when your workout starts to feel easy. Keeping that in mind, this program comes with progression built in. In the first 3 weeks, you'll learn the exercises using only bands. If you've never exercised with bands before or have never done any strength training, this will help you to get the hang of the movements, as well as how bands work. They can feel a little different from other types of strength-training equipment like machines or dumbbells when you try them for the first time. Unlike machines, which follow a set track, with bands there's nothing but your own muscles to guide the resistance through the right range of motion. That means it's important to go slowly and pay attention to your form. And unlike weights, bands get harder to lift the farther you stretch them, so you might need to experiment with where to hold the band.

Before you fear that you'll be slowing down your results by taking this incremental approach, here's a fun fact about exercising with bands. In a study run by *Prevention* magazine that compared weights, bands, balls, Pilates, yoga, and bodyweight-only exercises (like pushups), bands won hands down, helping exercisers who used them to shave off more pounds and inches than women who used any other type of equipment.

But back to the theme of progression: After 3 weeks you'll be ready to step it up to the next phase of the program—the double-duty combination exercises I've been so excited to share with you. The exercises will be the same movements you've been practicing for the first 3 weeks, but you'll add a dumbbell by holding the band and dumbbell together in your hand, or—in one move—even squeezing a dumbbell behind your knee (tricky!). At this point, you can continue to do these exercises for the remainder of the program if you like, keeping the challenge up by boosting the size of your dumbbell or increasing the resistance of the bands (see "Helpful Hints: The Incredible Adaptable Band" on page 26 for ways to tweak the resistance up or down using bands). And don't worry: Throughout this book I'll be reminding you to check whether you're pushing yourself at the appropriate level for you.

Bored and ready for some new moves? By the final weeks of this program you may be ready for a new challenge. That's why we created "Make It Harder" versions of the already hardworking exercises from this book. These moves will continue to build that fat-melting strength while adding new challenges—balancing on one foot while doing the move, for example—to keep things interesting and tone additional muscles.

Why Cardio Still Matters

You may be thinking by now that cardio is an afterthought in this program. Far from it! Studies have found that—total minutes per week being equal—cardio and strength exercise combined are better than either one alone. In one study from the prestigious *Journal of the American Medical*

Association, researcher Timothy S. Church, MD, PhD, MPH, and his colleagues at the Pennington Biomedical Research Center in Baton Rouge, Louisiana, had 262 men and women embark on one of four plans: no exercise; three long cardio workouts a week; three resistance exercise sessions a week; or three shorter cardio workouts supplemented with two strength workouts that added up to the same amount of time spent by the other exercise groups who did one or the other type of workout. While all of the exercise groups managed to shave inches from their waistlines, the folks who did both strength and cardio workouts lost 20 percent more weight. And perhaps the most outstanding result: The members of the group that combined strength and cardio were the only ones to see increases in their oxygen capacity (an indication of improved aerobic fitness that helps you to exercise harder while huffing and puffing less) as well as improved markers of blood sugar control, helping to manage diabetes risk.

So cardio is still an essential part of this program. But we didn't choose just any cardio exercise. Like the strength-training example above, you may have been doing cardio for years and don't understand why you're not seeing better results. In fact, some of the women on our test panel had already been walking most days of the week and still found themselves overweight at the start of the study. (Don't worry—if you love walking, you can still walk for exercise on this program. We're just going to teach you how to do it more effectively.) Adding muscle through our strength-training program is a good start, as we've already talked about. But taking a new, smarter approach to cardio can help you get better results in less time. Yes, you read that right!

In fact, you can shorten your workout time by 76 percent and get even better results—better results to the tune of boosting fat metabolism (the rate at which your body burns fat) by one-third in as little as 2 weeks of this type of training. Not to mention that the types of workouts we've included in the cardio chapter of this book keep the calorie burn higher once you're done, so as many as 120 bonus calories pull a disappearing act after you move on to the next thing on your to-do list.

The magic ingredient is intensity. Sounds hard, I know. And you're right—it will challenge you more than a casual window-shopping stroll.

HEAD-TO-TOE TONING SNACK

One of my favorite research findings on strength training—and one that's been replicated in a handful of different studies in recent years—is that chocolate milk is a perfect postworkout snack to help you rehydrate, refuel, and even build more lean muscle. In fact, a paper presented at the annual meeting of the American College of Sports Medicine reported that exercisers who sipped chocolate milk after working out shifted twice as much fat to muscle (including 2.5 times greater fat-to-muscle shift in their midsections) compared with those who drank a traditional carb-based sports drink. That's right, it's the one time that chocolate is an ideal get-fit food, thanks to a perfect blend of carbohydrates and protein. So I asked Tracy Gensler, the registered dietitian who developed the eating plan in this book, to create a special chocolate milk recipe that would fit this plan. It turned out that Ovaltine chocolate drink mix (my favorite!) fit best, because its lower sugar content allowed us to drink enough milk to hit our protein goal plus make the milk nice and chocolaty without going overboard on calories. Simply mix 1¼ cups fat-free milk with 4 tablespoons Ovaltine, and aim to drink it within an hour of your workout for the maximum effect.

But the trick is that you don't have to keep it up as long. By alternating bursts of power-walking (or whatever is your aerobic exercise of choice) with bouts at a slowed-down pace—a method called interval training—you increase the size and number of your mitochondria, the little powerhouses in your cells that use oxygen to convert calories and fat to usable energy. The resulting beefed-up muscle capacity means that you burn more calories and fat even while you sleep.

Eating for Energy—And Weight Loss

If you've gotten this far, but you're worried that all this exercise is going to leave you so famished you'll end up gaining weight, I have news for you. There are actually a number of reasons that exercise in general, and this program specifically, will help you to regulate your weight even more effectively than if you didn't exercise. First of all, while everyone's body is a little different, research has found that the very types of workouts included in this plan may actually help to quell your appetite—not increase it. Scientists at the University of Loughborough in Leicestershire, England, compared levels of the hormone ghrelin (a hormone that stimulates hunger) and peptide YY (a hormone that dampens hunger) following a variety of different workouts. Turns out that strength training decreased the ghrelin and running both boosted peptide YY and lowered ghrelin levels for a double dose of improved appetite control.

It may come as a shock that what you eat has more to do with your brain and hormone levels than those oh-so-hard-to-resist cravings for chocolate. After all, those office birthday cakes can pose quite the temptation even if you just ate lunch. But it turns out that cravings might be a bit more complex than you give them credit for.

In fact, there's a fascinating body of research spanning half a century that looks at the differences in how closely active and inactive people regulate the number of calories they eat compared with the number they burn. Back in the 1950s, researchers studied the caloric intake of a group of mill workers in India. They found that the men who had more laborious jobs ate almost exactly the number of calories they burned through the day. The sedentary workers, on the other hand, tended to eat much more than they burned.

More recently, researchers have examined this discrepancy in more controlled settings. The scenario goes like this: The subjects come into the lab and are given a drink while they fill out paperwork describing their physical activity habits. Then, to thank them for their participation, they are invited to an all-you-can-eat lunch buffet. Unbeknownst to the subjects, the researchers are secretly watching and weighing, keeping track of how much they eat. But guess what: There's another twist. Some of the subjects were given high-calorie sugary drinks, while others were given low-calorie, artificially sweetened drinks. Similar to the hardworking West Bengal mill workers back in the 1950s, the active subjects had an innate sense of what their body needed and adjusted their serving sizes at lunch depending on which drink they'd been given. If they'd sipped extra calories before lunch, they ate a little less from the buffet. If they had been given a diet drink, they increased the amount they ate. The sedentary subjects, on the other hand, had no built-in fuel gauge. They ate roughly the same amount regardless of which drink they were given.

Think exercisers are just born that way? The lab coats thought of that, too, so for the latest study they took sedentary participants, did the tests, and then put them on a 6-week exercise program before repeating the test. The second time around, the newly minted exercisers had sharpened their fuel gauges, eating an amount in line with their calorie needs. Pretty cool, huh?

There are ways that your diet can help you lose weight, though, and it's not just about eating less. Eating the right foods at the right times helps make sure you have both the energy to give your workouts your all and the nutrients your body needs to grow strong and toned. For example, getting enough protein—something that women tend to fall short on, especially as we get older and focus less on sitting down to "real" meals—is key to building those lean, sculpted muscles. While there's no protein powder on this plan, the meals and snacks are designed to provide at least 15 grams of protein within an hour of your strength workouts, something that's been shown to boost strength gains by as much as 63 percent.

Finally, while in general I'm a believer in gradual weight loss—it's safe, it tends to mean losing less lean muscle tissue, and it's easier to maintain than crash dieting—nothing is more motivating than seeing weight come off. That's why we created the Lighten-Up 7-Day Kickstart Menu to launch the program. This special week of meals has slightly fewer calories than the rest of the program, but because the workouts in Week 1 are focused on learning the exercises and getting into a groove rather than anything too strenuous, it's fitting. The main focus this week, though, is on keeping your sodium low and your potassium high—two dietary minerals that work together to regulate water retention (read: bloated or not). By ridding yourself of excess water weight this first week, you'll feel refreshed, energized, and ready to rock for Weeks 2 through 8.

Now, let's get started!

Merry Buckley

Age 39

Lost: 11 pounds and 6.5 inches

Gained: 20 percent more strength in her upper and lower body

Favorite exercise: "The Lunge Repeaters. My thighs are so much more toned than before, thanks to this move I love to hate!"

Merry Buckley had watched herself gradually gaining a pound a year since college. "I hadn't gained lots of weight since college, but I had lost muscle mass and gained fat, and I could tell that my strength had declined," she says. At age 39, she was "determined to halt the march to porkiness" when she heard about the Tone Every Inch program from a friend. Starting off, she decided she'd be thrilled to lose any weight—ideally about 10 pounds—but she'd be happy just learning how to stop the gain. Her biggest challenge: time. With 5-year-old and 6-year-old sons, her days are split between working as a writer and coordinating carpools. "I don't mind working hard," she says, "but I hate taking a lot of time to get exercise done."

Like several other members of our test panel, Merry already was a fairly regular exerciser. In fact, she even did a couple miles of jogging mixed with walking about three times a week, biked occasionally when the weather behaved, and lifted weights from time to time. But she wasn't seeing the results she wanted. Until now. After 3 weeks on the Tone Every Inch program, Merry was already almost 6 pounds lighter, and at the end of 8 weeks she had surpassed her weight loss goal with a pound to spare. Top it off with a 12 percent reduction in body fat, and Merry is looking fitter from head to toe. Her favorite new-and-improved body part? Her lower back, the site of the former cursed fat pockets above the butt and below the bra strap that plague so many women as they get older. And let's not forget a set of sexy, sculpted legs that look better than ever in a skirt—and are powerful enough to lift 20 percent more weight than when she started. "I was already running and biking before all this," she says, "and my legs didn't look like this!"

Focusing on getting enough protein in her diet was another revelation for Merry, who considered herself to be a healthy eater but had never focused carefully on what she ate. Prioritizing the protein that would help her to preserve precious muscle mass as she lost weight had the side effect of staving off the afternoon slump. "I'd never really paid attention to how much protein was in my daily diet, and it took a little effort to make sure I was getting it in there, but I was surprised at how full I felt by the end of the day despite cutting back on calories." Not a big fan of cooking meat, Merry has learned how to prepare beans, tofu, and tempeh. "And I love quinoa," she says of the high-protein ricelike grain.

Merry's only regret is that she didn't do this sooner. "It was startlingly easy once I got started to use just a little self-discipline, complete the exercises each week, and stick with the calorie guidelines. I've made these sustainable changes to my lifestyle by eating better and exercising smarter, and I'm continuing to lose weight," she says. "I don't have a goal in mind because I'm not sure where it's going to end up. I'm just different now and my body is changing."

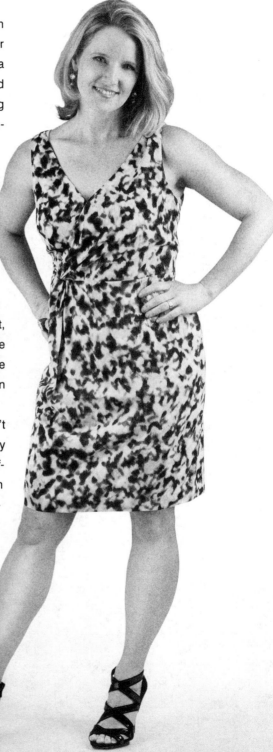

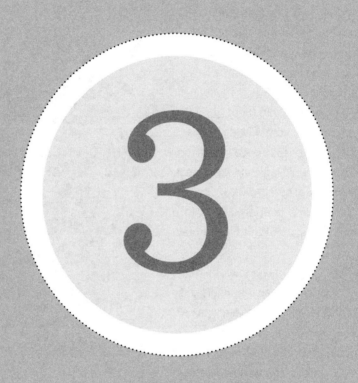

All About Bands

Bands are a home exerciser's best friend. They're small and inexpensive, and they allow you to do everything you could do with a big weight machine at the gym for a fraction of the price (or shelling out for monthly gym fees) and without dedicating a room in your house to working out. And above all, they work—arguably more so than those pricey space hogs because bands offer more "functional" training that mimics real-life movements. Our test panelists were fans, too: "I love the bands. Especially as you get older, they seem more joint-friendly," says Barbara Terrell, 54. "They definitely have made me feel stronger, but also more flexible than free weights ever have." For tester Colleen Barnes, 47, the tension of the bands keeps her focused on the whole movement, not just throwing a dumbbell up and down.

Whether you've never used resistance bands before or you want to learn to use them more effectively, the first part of this program will give you a chance to get the hang of working out with bands and "dust off the cobwebs" (as Tone Every Inch tester Sherri Dunham described it) as you start to tone and tighten those metabolism-maximizing muscles.

Welcome to Band Camp

Although these exercises are a warmup for the combination band-and-dumbbell exercises that will come in Chapter 4, don't think for a second that this is a lesser workout! When *Prevention* magazine compared the effects of a resistance band workout similar to this one with workouts based on other equipment like stability balls and weights, the bands blew away the competition, helping testers to lose as many as 14 pounds (18 percent more than the runner-up routine) and trimming up to 9 inches from their waistlines (a boost of nearly one-third compared to other workouts) in 12 weeks. Not bad for something you can stick in your purse!

In fact, that portability may be the best feature of bands—they can go anywhere with you. When tester Colleen Barnes jetted off to Costa Rica to chaperone her stepdaughter's school trip in the middle of the program, she packed her bands and kept up with the program just like she would have at home. "Eating well on vacation is always tough—though rice and beans offered at every meal made it easier. The bands, on the other hand, were no problem to use away from home. I had to forgo the weights for a week, but it was great to at least get the band exercises in."

While I'd love to believe that there's some magic ingredient in resistance bands that makes them so superior, it may be as simple as the fact that they're easier to have on hand so there are no excuses, just results. They're as simple to use in your living room, bedroom, or even hotel room as they are at the gym, translating to fewer skipped workouts. And fewer missed sessions mean more pounds and inches—*poof*—gone.

But don't get me wrong—bands do have a few standout features that help them to do their sculpting job so effectively. They offer a smoother and more consistent challenge for your muscles than dumbbells do, because when you lift something weighted like a dumbbell, it feels heaviest only during a small part of the exercise, explains Gary Sforzo, PhD, the exercise physiologist and Ithaca College professor of exercise science whose original study inspired this book. And you can make subtle adjustments even as you do the exercise to make it more or less challenging, for example, by choking up on the band to shorten the

⤵ Helpful Hints: The Incredible Adaptable Band

One of my favorite features of bands is their ability to meet you where you are strengthwise. Unlike dumbbells, which jump in standard increments that can sometimes leave you between two weights, bands can truly be adjusted almost infinitely. Here's how:

Choke up/down. The most basic of adjustments, this can be done on the fly even midexercise. The closer you hold the band to its anchor, the harder you'll have to pull to stretch it through the motion of the exercise. You can wrap it around your hand if you like, or just slide your grip up or down the band.

Use a lighter/heavier band. If you find the band is cutting into your hands, you're likely pulling too hard on a too-lax band. Bump up to the next resistance level. If you find you can't complete the full range of motion (for example, you can only get your forearm up to 90 degrees in a dumbbell curl rather than bringing the band all the way up to your shoulder), try a lighter band.

Widen/narrow your stance. If you're standing on the band with both feet, increasing or decreasing the length of band that's between your feet affects the length of working band that you have left to pull on. The shorter the length of band you're stretching in the exercise, the harder it will be.

Double it up. If you need a heavier resistance than the bands you currently have, stack them, using both at once for a single move.

length that you're stretching, or by releasing some of the band to lessen
the resistance (there are more tips on tweaking the resistance of your
band in "Helpful Hints: The Incredible Adaptable Band").

They can also be better for beginners than dumbbells. "Bands have
a softer, kinder feel," says Greg Niederlander, the director of products
(including elastic resistance) for Spri, a distributor of bands and other
fitness equipment. "Especially for a novice, bands can be safer because
the resistance increases gradually as you go through the movement,
slowing you down so you don't take the range of motion beyond where
you can safely go."

And because bands aren't gravity dependent like dumbbells, they
open up all-new movement options, says Niederlander, who in his 25
years at Spri has watched the rise in popularity of band workouts since
they first made their way from physical therapy into group fitness classes
in the early 1980s. Whereas dumbbells only provide resistance up and
down, bands allow you to work muscles in all different directions.

Setting the Stage

Whether you're doing the workout at a gym or in your living room, there
are just three things you need to do to get started. Here's a quick-start
guide:

○ **Choose your band.** The one piece of equipment you will need for this workout is a 5- to 6-foot resistance band, depending on your height. I'm 5-foot-8, and I prefer a 6-foot band, especially for moves that involve stretching the band all the way overhead. If you're shorter, a 5-foot band might be more comfortable and leave you with less excess to work with.

○ **Find a space.** You'll need enough room to spread your arms or legs wide in any direction without bumping into something. For the floor moves, you'll want to roll out an exercise mat (unless you have a carpeted floor you don't mind lying on for a couple of the moves).

○ **Select your anchor.** For some moves, you'll need to tie or loop the band around a sturdy object that won't move or slide when you pull on the band. See "Helpful Hints: Anchors Aweigh!" on page 53 for more on how to anchor your band.

➲ Helpful Hints: Less Is More

Listen up, overachievers: When the plan says to do 8 to 12 reps of each exercise, don't automatically read that as "Do 12 reps, unless you're a slacker." If you can dive right in and do 12 reps the first time through, chances are you need a firmer band. Start with a challenge that fatigues you in 8 reps and work on building up the number as you get stronger. Then it will be time to up the challenge again!

Band Exercises

Start warming up with about 5 minutes of easy cardio such as walking or marching in place. Add some forward and backward arm circles, and rotate your torso to the right and left as you walk to get your upper body loosened up as well. Then start the first move. Do each exercise 8 to 12 times, or 8 to 12 times per side where relevant. This will be one set. Without stopping for longer than it takes to transition (unless you need to), go on to the next exercise, or repeat the exercise on the opposite side if needed. Do all 10 moves, then come back and repeat the sequence if you're doing a second or third set.

If you find that a move is too challenging at first, try the "Make It Easier" variation. Many of these options simplify the exercise by separating a combined movement (which is more efficient once you get the hang of it) into two separate exercises (which can be easier to figure out when you're starting out). A major component of strength training is strengthening the neuromuscular system, or the connections between the brain and the muscles necessary to coordinate a movement—and to push or pull against a resistance you're not used to. Don't worry; these nervous system adaptations happen quickly—even faster than you'll gain any actual muscle strength—so you'll be up to speed in no time.

① Two-Way Row

(feel it in your: arms and shoulders)

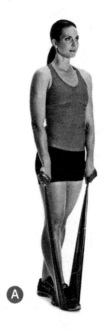

A

Step 1. Stand with your feet staggered, right foot forward, with the middle of the band secured under your right foot, ends in either hand (Photo A).

Step 2. Palms facing back, bend your elbows out to the sides, stretching the band up until your hands are about chest height (Photo B).

Step 3. Pause, then slowly lower to the starting position.

Step 4. Repeat, this time turning your wrists so your palms face in toward your sides and your elbows point back as you pull up (Photo C). Continue alternating directions for 8 to 12 total reps (each pull counts as 1 rep), and switch the forward foot after each set.

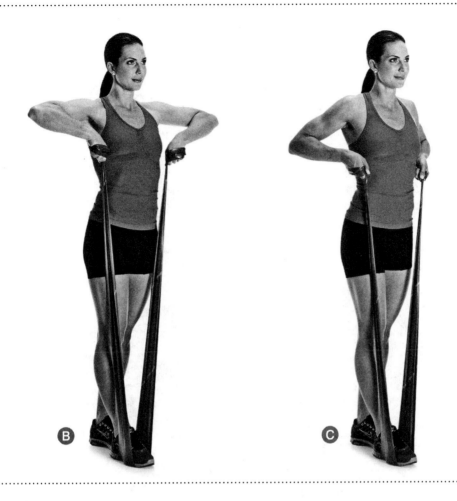

B

C

➡ *Make It Easier*

Do the move with one arm at a time. This will allow you to focus more carefully on good form without having to coordinate two separate movements and, if you need it, will allow you to create more slack in the band, which lightens the resistance.

➡ *Faster Toning Tip*

Make sure to keep your shoulders down so they don't inch their way up toward your ears, creating tension in your neck. When you lift with your palms facing your sides and your elbows pointing back, imagine your shoulder blades drawing toward each other.

② Pickup and Shrug

(feel it in your: shoulders, lower back, butt, and back of thighs)

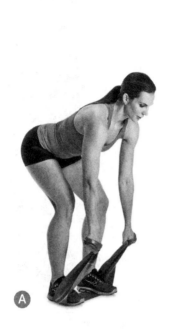

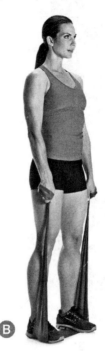

Step 1. Stand with your feet hip-width apart, band under both feet, one end gripped in each hand.

Step 2. Keeping your abs tight to support your back, bend your knees slightly and stick your butt back as you hinge from your hips, bending forward until your back is nearly parallel with the floor (Photo A).

Step 3. Choke up on the band (gather the excess in your hands or wind it around your hands) so it's taut, then squeeze your glutes (butt) to lift your torso back to standing (Photo B).

Step 4. Shrug your shoulders up toward your ears (Photo C), then lower them and repeat for 8 to 12 reps to complete a set.

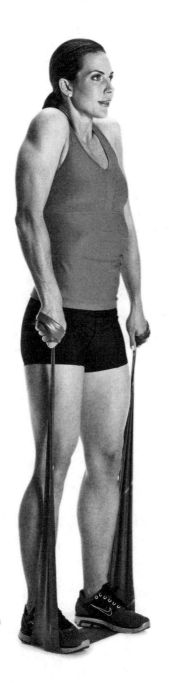

C

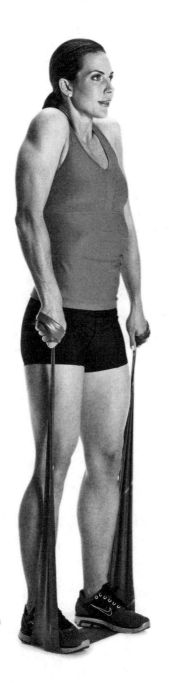

➡ *Make It Easier*

Release some of the band so it's not as taut at the beginning of the move and only hinge forward as far as you can while maintaining good posture.

➡ *Faster Toning Tip*

Focus on your posture with this move. Imagine there's a broomstick strapped to your back, keeping it stable throughout the move. Keep your chest lifted and shoulder blades pulled back, and make sure not to round your back.

③ Chest Press

(feel it in your: chest and arms)

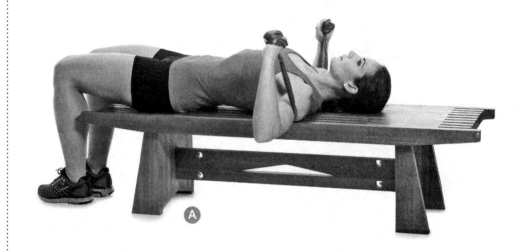

Ⓐ

Step 1. Lie on a bench if you have one (a coffee table can also work), or on the floor if you don't, knees bent with feet flat on the floor. Position the band under your upper back with one end in either hand near your underarms, elbows bent (Photo A).

Step 2. Stretch the band up toward the ceiling until your arms are straight but not locked (Photo B).

Step 3. Pause, then slowly return to the starting position. Repeat for 8 to 12 reps to complete 1 set.

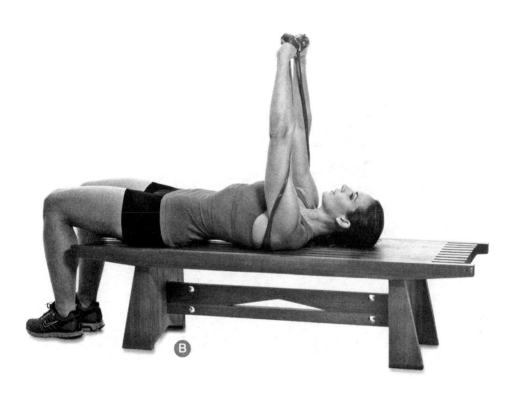

Make It Easier

Use a lighter band or slide your hands toward the ends of the band.

Faster Toning Tip

Keep your shoulders down and away from your ears.

4
Side Leg-Lift Crunch

(feel it in your: hips, butt, and obliques)

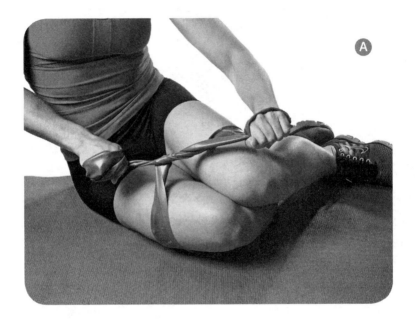

Step 1. Securely tie a resistance band snugly around both legs above your knees (Photo A).

Step 2. Lie on your right side with your right arm stretched out in front, legs stacked, and your left arm bent with your elbow toward the ceiling and your left fingers by your ear (Photo B).

Step 3. Simultaneously raise your top leg while crunching your torso up (Photo C).

Step 4. Pause, then lower your torso and leg to the starting position. Repeat for 8 to 12 reps, then switch sides to complete 1 set.

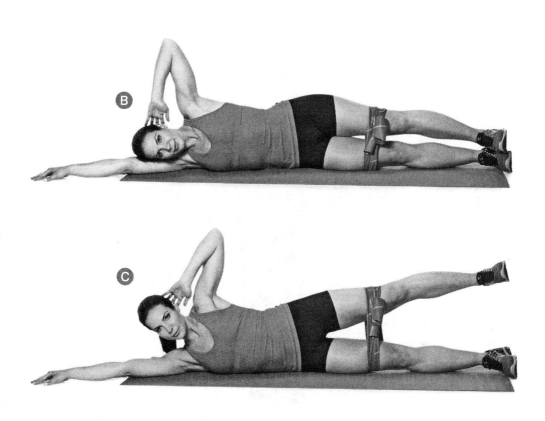

➡ *Make It Easier*

Separate the exercise into two moves: side leg lifts and side crunches. Once you get the hang of each movement individually, put them back together.

➡ *Faster Toning Tip*

Imagine your body is sandwiched between two panes of glass. Try to keep your body in a straight line between the panes as you lift your torso and your leg so you don't touch the glass.

⑤ Cheerleader Press

(feel it in your: shoulders, arms, and triceps)

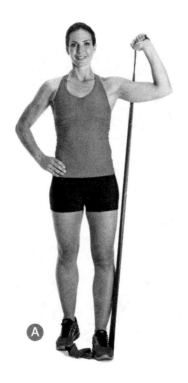

Ⓐ

Step 1. Stand with your feet slightly staggered, left foot forward, one end of the band under your left foot and the free end gripped in your left hand (wrap the band around your hand if you have extra length). Bend your left elbow out to the side about 90 degrees at chest level (Photo A).

Step 2. Press your arm straight up overhead (Photo B). That's 1 rep.

Step 3. Bend your elbow to lower your forearm behind you (Photo C).

Step 4. Press upward again. That's 2 reps. Do 8 to 12 reps, then switch sides to complete a set.

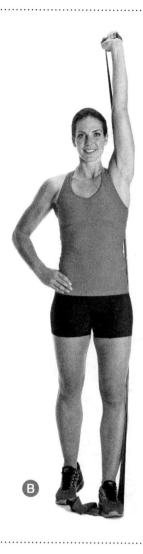

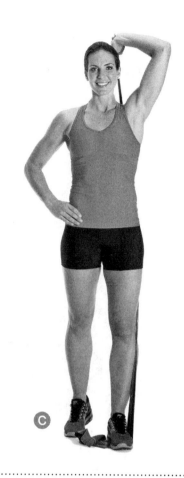

➡ *Make It Easier*

Break up the exercise into two moves: Do a set of 4 to 6 overhead presses (steps 1 and 2), then a set of 4 to 6 triceps extensions (steps 3 and 4). Once you're comfortable with the two moves separately, put them back together.

➡ *Faster Toning Tip*

To get the most upper-arm firming out of this move, try to keep your upper arm still as your forearm bends behind you and then presses back up.

6

Skater Side Twist

(feel it in your: hips, thighs, butt, and obliques)

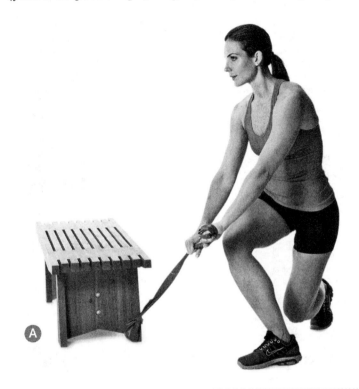

Step 1. Tie the band to a low, sturdy object like the leg of a piece of heavy furniture (see anchoring tips on page 53). Standing with the band anchored to your right, grasp the loose ends together in both hands, arms extended.

Step 2. Step diagonally back and to the right with your left foot, sitting back and bending your knees as though curtsying and reaching across your body toward the anchor point (Photo A).

Step 3. Stand, toes pointing forward, and rotate your torso away from the band anchor (Photo B). Repeat for 8 to 12 reps, then switch sides to complete 1 set.

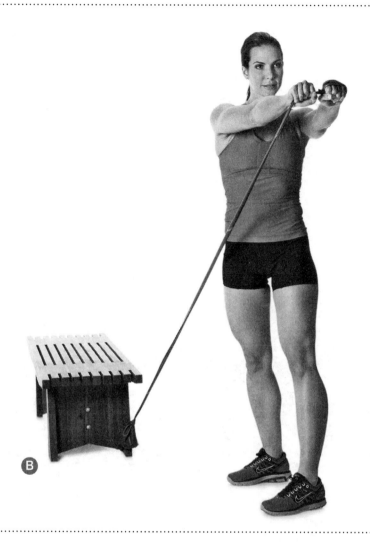

B

➡ **Make It Easier**

Don't bend your knees as deeply into the curtsy lunge.

➡ **Faster Toning Tip**

To protect your knees while doing this move, make sure your knees and toes are always pointing in the same direction.

Pullover and Crunch

(feel it in your: triceps and abs)

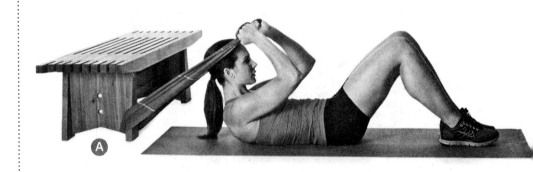

Ⓐ

Step 1. Loop the band around a sturdy object like the leg of a piece of heavy furniture. Lie on your back with your head in front of the anchored band, knees bent, and feet flat on the floor. Bending your elbows, reach back to grasp one end of the band in each hand, hands near your ears.

Step 2. Engage your abs to crunch upward (Photo A).

Step 3. Without lowering your body, straighten your elbows and extend your arms forward (Photo B).

Step 4. Slowly lower your body, then your arms, back to the starting position. Do 8 to 12 reps to complete a set.

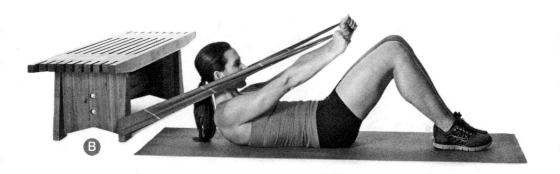

B

➡️ *Make It Easier*

Slide closer to the band's anchor point to relax the tension in the band.

➡️ *Faster Toning Tip*

To maximize firming in the backs of your upper arms (aka the chicken wings), try to keep your upper arms stationary as you straighten your elbows to press your forearms forward.

8

Lunge Repeater

(feel it in your: arms, butt, hips, thighs, and legs)

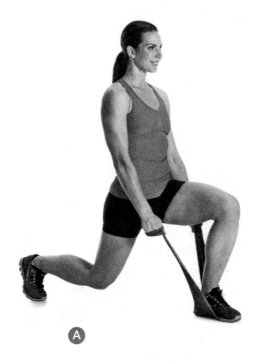

A

Step 1. Stand with your feet hip-width apart, the center of the band under your left foot. Hold one end of the band in each hand, arms at sides, palms facing in.

Step 2. Take a big step backward with your right leg, bending both knees to lower into a lunge with your left knee directly over your ankle (Photo A).

Step 3. Bend your elbows, curling your hands toward your shoulders, palms facing in (Photo B).

Step 4. Step forward to stand (Photo C). Slowly lower your arms. Do 8 to 12 reps per side to complete a set.

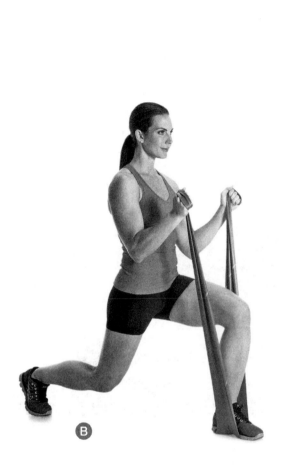

(B)

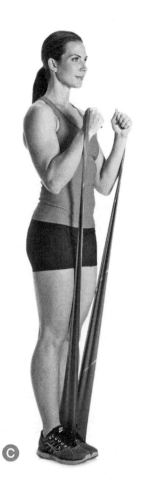

(C)

➡ *Make It Easier*

Keep your feet planted in a split stance rather than stepping into and out of the lunge. Simply bend your knees to lower, curl your arms up, then straighten your knees without stepping forward to stand.

➡ *Faster Toning Tip*

Timing is key to getting the most out of this move. Make sure you keep your hands curled up toward your shoulders until you've returned to standing in order to maximize thigh and butt toning.

9

Butt Kicker

(feel it in your: butt, backs of thighs, and abs)

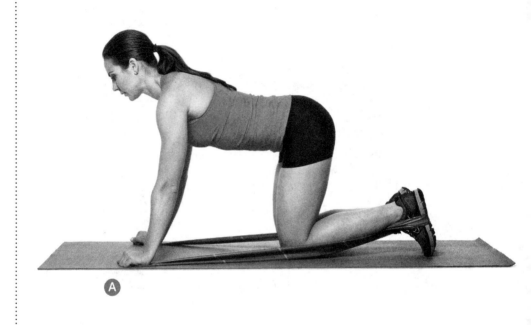

Ⓐ

Step 1. Get into a tabletop position on your hands and knees, wrists directly below your shoulders and knees below your hips. Wrap the band around your left heel, crisscross the two sides of the band, and grasp one end in each hand (Photo A).

Step 2. Keeping your right foot flexed and knee bent, press your left heel up and back (Photo B). Repeat 8 to 12 times to complete a set, then switch legs and repeat.

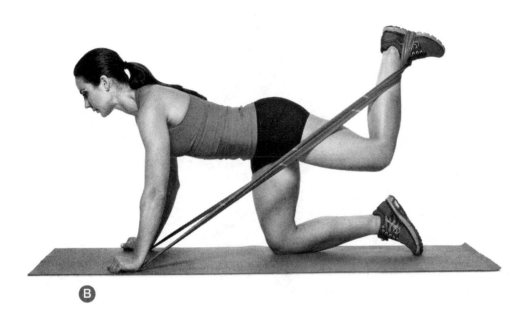

Ⓑ

➡ *Make It Easier*

Practice the exercise
without the band if needed
until you get the hang of it.
Then add the band to
boost the challenge.

➡ *Faster Toning Tip*

To avoid neck or back
strain—and to get a bit of
bonus core strength from
this move—keep your neck
in line with your spine, your
back flat, and your abs
pulled up and in as you do
this exercise.

⑩
Squat and Curl

(feel it in your: butt, thighs, and arms)

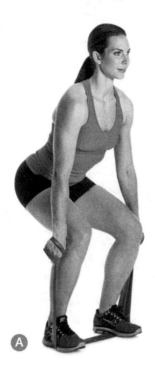

Ⓐ

Step 1. Stand with your feet hip-width apart, the band under both feet, a loose end in each hand.

Step 2. Bend your knees to sit back, keeping your knees behind your toes (Photo A).

Step 3. With your palms facing your sides, bend your elbows to curl your forearms upward, rotating your palms to face your chest (Photo B).

Step 4. Press into your heels to stand (Photo C), then lower your arms to the starting position. Do 8 to 12 reps to complete a set.

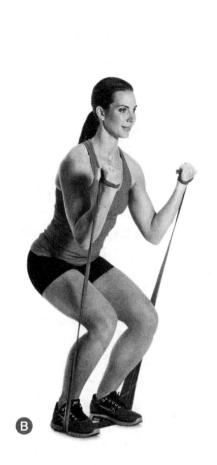

B

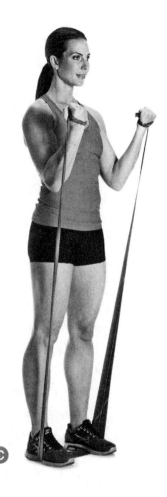

C

➡ *Make It Easier*

Follow the squat progression in the box on pages 50–51.

➡ *Faster Toning Tip*

Keep your upper arms glued to your sides as you curl your forearms up toward your shoulders, and make sure not to reverse the movement until you've risen out of the squat position.

THREE STEPS TO MASTERING THE NUMBER ONE BUTT BLASTER

If doing squats feels like the equivalent of one of those blind-trust team-building experiments—you know, the one where you fall backward and "trust" somebody to catch you—you might be tempted to erase them from your repertoire in exchange for safer-feeling exercises. Don't do it!

When polled by the American Council on Exercise (ACE), a panel of personal trainers voted squats the hands-down best all-around butt exercise. In fact, when ACE did a follow-up study using electromyographic (EMG) analysis to actually measure the muscle activation in the gluteus maximus (butt), gluteus medius (hips), and hamstrings (backs of the thighs), the squat was the yardstick against which all eight exercises in the study were measured. The result? Squats kept their crown as the best butt-beautifier, but shared it with another move on this plan: butt kickers.

And it's not just about a perky derriere. The butt happens to be the biggest muscle in your body, giving it a ton of metabolic potential. Using more muscle means you burn more calories while you're doing the exercise, and the strength you develop will help you keep burning more calories afterward. Squats also target the fronts of your thighs, or your quadriceps, as well as the many smaller muscles that surround and support your knees, helping to ward off osteoarthritis and knee injuries. So now that I've (I hope) convinced you not to skip squats, let's learn some modifications that may make them more comfortable as you build up the balance and strength to do them safely and effectively.

Level 1: Wall sits. Stand with your feet shoulder-width apart, 1 to 2 feet in front of a wall. Place your back against the wall. Bend your knees, sliding your back down the wall, aiming to lower until both your knees and your hips are bent to about 90 degrees, with your knees over your ankles and behind your toes (Photo A). Hold for up to a minute. When you've gotten the hang of it, add the band, securing it under both feet. Curl your arms up toward your shoulders and complete all the reps of the arm curls while holding the lower-body position (take a break midway if you need to).

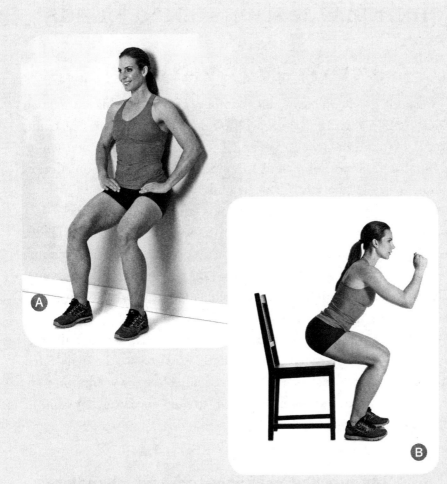

Level 2: Wall squats. Get into position like you did in Level 1, but this time do repetitions, pressing into your heels to slide back up the wall to stand, then lowering again. Do all your reps sliding back up and down the wall. When you're ready, add the band and do the Squat and Curl move from page 48 with your back against the wall.

Level 3: Chair squats. Step away from the wall and stand in front of a sturdy chair or bench. Bend your knees to sit back and lightly touch your rear to the seat before immediately standing up (Photo B). When you're comfortable with the squat portion of the move, add the bands and arm curls. Work toward sitting until you almost touch, but not quite; once you can do that, you're ready to ditch the chair.

Common Questions about Bands

Q Where can I buy resistance bands?

A Bands are available at just about any sporting goods store (such as Dick's or Sports Authority), as well as many department and discount stores (I've found them at Target and T.J. Maxx). The flat bands, which I prefer for this workout, tend to come in packs of three different resistance levels and usually cost around $10.

However, in my experience these bands tend to be on the short side—about 4 feet long, while I recommend more like 5 or 6 feet. The longer length is helpful if you're taller, as well as for the exercises that involve reaching the band all the way from the floor to overhead. For longer bands, you'll likely have more luck online. For the trial run of this program, we used Resist-A-Bands available from Spri (www.spriproducts.com), which come in 5-foot bands in a variety of resistance levels as well as 6-yard bulk rolls of band that can be cut to your desired length. We also used the Dyna-Band brand, which offers 6-foot lengths of band, available at www.amazon.com. They may be more durable—and less likely to snap—because they come in wider widths than most.

Q My gym has resistance tubes with handles. Can I do the workout with these?

A Absolutely. Resistance tubing offers the same benefits as flat bands, and they even tend to be more durable. That's why you're likely to see tubing in most gyms, where they see heavy use. The reason I prefer flat bands for this workout (and in general) is because I consider one of the best things about bands to be the ability to change the resistance by changing the length of the band. Handles that stay in a fixed position make it harder to do this. An easy way around this is to simply ignore the handles and hold the band directly at whatever length you need it to be for the exercise. You may find the loose handles to be annoying or

➲ Helpful Hints: Anchors Aweigh!

Some exercises require you to secure an end or the middle of the band to an object sturdy enough to pull against without moving it. It may take some experimentation to find a good spot to anchor your band, but once you figure out what works in your home, you'll be good to go. Here are a few suggestions to get you started.

Tie or loop it to a furniture leg. My go-to band anchor is usually the leg of a piece of furniture. I've successfully used a bedpost or the foot of an antique trunk at the end of my bed as well as my coffee table and couch legs in the living room. While

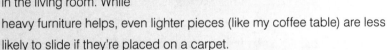

heavy furniture helps, even lighter pieces (like my coffee table) are less likely to slide if they're placed on a carpet.

Knot it in the door. Another method if your furniture just doesn't do the trick: the door. Simply tie a knot (or two) in your band and shut it at the correct height in the door so the knot is on the outside of the door and the loose end(s) of the band are on your side. Just make sure nobody's going to open the door midexercise!

Buy a door anchor. This simple band accessory (I bought one from Thera-Band for less than $5 on www .amazon.com) follows a similar principle to the knot-tying technique above, minus the knots to tie and untie. Simply slip it into your door and you have a plastic disk on one side of the door to hold things tight, and a loop on the other side to pass your band through.

in the way at first, but I guarantee you'll get used to it within a couple of workouts and figure out a technique that works for you.

Q I don't want to bulk up. Should I stick to lighter resistance bands and do more reps?

A Using resistance bands that are too light to challenge your muscles is more likely to undermine your results than it is to prevent bulk. You have heard this before, but it bears repeating: No matter what size bands you lift, as a woman you're simply not at risk of ending up looking like the Incredible Hulk. That's because you have far less testosterone, a hormone necessary for creating significant bulk, than superheroes, male body builders, or the typical man. Sure, you can lift lighter weights for more repetitions, but rather than creating less bulk, you'll most likely just gain less strength and muscle and see more limited results from this program.

Need proof? In a study by researchers at Central Michigan University in Mount Pleasant, women worked the biceps in one arm by doing three sets of five arm curls with heavy weights. With the other arm, they lifted lighter weights 24 times in a row. The total amount of weight was matched so both arms lifted the same amounts. For example, if the right arm lifted 5 pounds 24 times, or a total of 120 pounds, the left arm lifted 8 pounds 15 times, which also totaled 120 pounds. Turned out, the heavy lifters gained 55 percent more metabolism-revving strength in 10 weeks, yet both arms remained the exact same size. Another reason to go heavy: Research has shown that total pounds lifted being equal, hoisting a heavy weight fewer times gives your calorie burn a 25 percent bigger boost than lifting less weight for more reps.

Q How far can my band safely stretch?

A I checked with Greg Niederlander, the director of products for Spri, on this one because he's the resistance band pro. High-quality bands, like Resist-A-Band (which Spri sells) or Dyna-Band, should stretch to about 2.5 to 3 times their original length. You'll know if a band has been stretched too far or is losing its elasticity if you notice that it's starting to turn white. To gauge when a band's at the end of its life, you should also examine it regularly, looking for holes or tears in the rubber.

Q. **When I do exercises with the bands, I don't feel like my muscles are being challenged like they are when I lift dumbbells. What gives?**

A. There are two likely culprits at play: either the band you're using or your form (or both). If you are using a band that's too light, your muscles aren't getting the resistance they need to adapt and grow stronger. Remember that, since resistance bands are often used for rehab and physical therapy, you will probably never need the lightest band available. Those are for people coming back from injuries. Luckily, it's an easy enough fix by swapping yours for a more resistive band.

When it comes to form, there are a couple of areas to troubleshoot. Start with how you're holding the band. Is it taut at the beginning of the move? If not, when you stretch the band throughout the exercise's range of motion, you won't be getting any resistance at all (or very little). Choking up on the band or wrapping it around your hand a couple of times should help. The next thing to address is your speed. If you're flying through reps—especially with a light band—your momentum is likely doing the work. (Think about a car rolling down the street. How much of a difference would it make if you got behind it and started pushing?) As you perform each exercise, go slow and focus on how your muscle is engaging against the resistance of the band.

Q. **How do I know if my band is too difficult for me?**

A. Kudos to you for not being afraid to push yourself! You'll know the band you're using is too heavy if you can't complete the full range of motion of the exercise (for example, you can bend your arm to only

90 degrees when trying to do a biceps curl instead of bringing your hand all the way up to your shoulder. If you are using the full length of the band and you can't do even close to 8 reps, save that band for when you're a little stronger.

Keeping Track of Your Workouts

Knowing how many sets and reps you did in your last workout and how much resistance you used for each exercise is a helpful reminder when it's time to grab the right band for your next workout. It helps you to see when you might be ready to jump to the next level of band (for example, if you've been doing several sets of 12 reps for a few workouts in a row). And it serves as a good checklist to make sure you don't forget any moves.

Women who write down their workouts also exercise more each week and lose more weight overall when compared with those who simply do it and forget it. This finding comes from a study in the *Journal of the American Dietetic Association,* for which researchers examined 20 years' worth of studies on various types of self-monitoring among dieters and exercisers. In one of the reviewed studies, the most consistent self-monitors lost almost twice as much as inconsistent peers—an average of 23 pounds compared with just 12 pounds for those who didn't fill out their logs regularly. The regular loggers also accrued nearly twice as much exercise—an average of 174 minutes a week versus 89 minutes for nonloggers. See a sample log at right. For a blank log page you can copy and use, flip to page 306 in the Tone Every Inch Logs.

Band Workout Log

Week of program: (2) **Date:** _3/11/12_

EXERCISE	REPS	WEIGHT USED (COLOR OF BAND)	OBSERVATIONS/ CHALLENGES
Two-Way Row	10/8	Green band	
Pickup and Shrug	12/11	Blue band	
Chest Press	10/10	Blue band	
Side Leg-Lift Crunch	12/10	Green band	
Cheerleader Press	12/12	Orange band	Use green next time
Skater Side Twist	12/12	Blue band	
Pullover and Crunch	10/8	Green band	
Lunge Repeater	12/10	Blue band	Next time add orange band
Butt Kicker	12/12	Green band	Use blue next time
Squat and Curl	12/10	Blue band	

Sherri Dunham

Age 45

Lost: 4 inches and 4 pounds of fat

Gained: More positive energy, confidence, motivation, and all-around oomph!

Favorite newly sculpted body part: Her arms

Time and convenience have always been the trickiest exercise hurdles for 45-year-old Sherri Dunham. She used to love going to kickboxing and step aerobics classes until her lunch hour was changed to 1:00 p.m. and there weren't any classes that fit her new schedule. As a result, despite near-daily walking, she could feel herself losing muscle, gradually adding weight, and generally feeling "frumpy." When she saw an online posting at work for the Tone Every Inch program, it seemed like the perfect way to jump-start herself into just doing something.

"I was really at a stagnant point," Sherri says, "but I'm not one to just go and use machines." She missed the structure of having an instructor telling her exactly what to do, and without that she felt lost. Besides, machines are just boring, she says. Having a plan of action gave her the confidence to go to the gym solo, and she learned how something as simple as chatting with and getting to know the gym staff could add the social element she had loved about classes—while she could work around her own schedule.

By Week 3 Sherri was down almost 4 pounds, and she finished the 8 weeks with a reduction of nearly 8 percent body fat. "When I wear a sleeveless shirt now, I'm like, 'Holy cow, what happened to the lump hanging there?'" she jokes. Her husband likes to compliment her "big guns," though Sherri is quick to clarify that they're not huge. (Our results confirm this; Sherri gained 2.75 pounds of muscle but lost inches from head to toe, especially in her hips and thighs, where she dropped nearly 4 inches.) She's also noticed a slimmer-in-pants waistline. "Since I had my twins (19 years ago), I felt like I had this belly fat I couldn't get rid of, and it feels tighter now," she says.

Sherri also noticed a big boost in feel-good energy as a by-product of exercising. "I don't feel as drained, I have a more posi-tive attitude, and I don't feel as grumpy looking in the mirror. I just feel better about myself," she explains. And she learned that every little bit helps. "I didn't find the time to do as much car-dio as I would have liked, but the study helped me see how adding even small amounts can make a big difference in your metabolism and every aspect of your health."

And she's not done yet. Next up with the twins home from college for vaca-tion, Sherri is looking forward to making workouts a family affair. With one son who is a football player, she's even con-sidering adding in some pushups to keep working on those awesome arms.

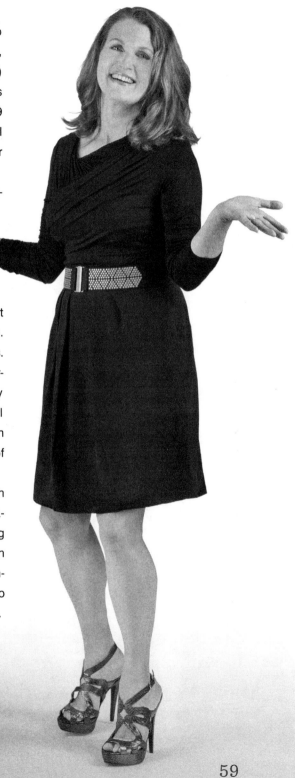

59

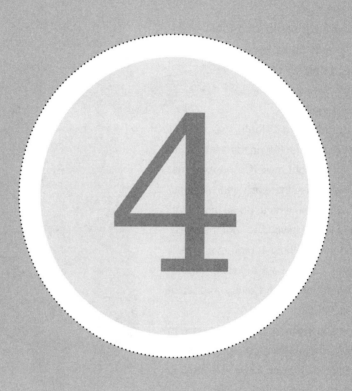

Time to Go Triple Time!

Now that you've mastered the band moves in Chapter 3, it's time for the main event. In this chapter, we'll take the same exercises you practiced for the first 3 weeks of the plan to the next level by adding a set of dumbbells. This super-sculpting exercise combo is what sets this plan apart from other routines you may have tried in the past.

That's because while ordinary strength training is certainly beneficial, in the Ithaca College study that inspired this program, this dumbbell-plus-band formula led to increases in both strength and power of up to three times that of exercisers who took a dumbbells-only approach in just 7 weeks of training. That is, exercisers who combined bands and weights increased the amount of weight they could hold while doing a squat by an average of more than 36 pounds, whereas peers who lifted dumbbells alone improved enough to lift only an additional 15 pounds. In the bench press, exercisers who paired weights and bands increased the amount they could lift by almost 15 pounds compared to just over 7 for the dumbbell-only crew. If that sounds like a lot of weight to lift, it's because the study subjects were college athletes (men and women) who already had several years of experience.

As a cherry on top, the combo exercisers gained triple the power, a measure of their strength combined with their speed, which researchers measured by how high they could jump at the beginning and end of the study. Power might sound like something that only matters to hardcore athletes, but it turns out it's especially valuable for women over 40. That's because it emphasizes type II, or fast twitch, muscles, which tend to be the first to go as you get older. Maintaining these type II fibers is one of the best ways to keep your metabolism humming at a youthful rate. Finally, the study subjects also gained more than twice as much lean muscle mass, helping them to burn calories and fat at a faster rate.

Putting the Weight in Weight Training

While researchers are still trying to understand what makes the band-plus-dumbbell combo so much more effective than traditional training, they do have some theories. For one, when you do an exercise with a dumbbell or a barbell, there's one small part of the move that is the most challenging. Exercise scientists dub this the sticking point, and it's typically the turnaround point of the exercise. For example, when you do a squat, the sticking point happens when you're at the lowest point of the exercise and you go to stand up. In an arm curl, the sticking point occurs when your arm is fully extended, and you first begin to curl the weight back up toward your shoulder. This so-called sticking point, then, places a limit on just how heavy a weight you can use for each exercise. Think of it this way: Even though you may be able to do 95 percent of an arm curl with a 10-pound dumbbell, if you can only get past that turnaround point while holding 5 pounds of weight, you'll have to stick to the 5-pound dumbbell for the whole exercise. (After all, you can't switch weights halfway through.)

Bands, on the other hand, have the opposite "sticking point." Because the band gets progressively more resistive the farther you stretch it, it's the hardest at the very top of the move. By stacking the two types of resistance together, you get a smoother, more consistent muscle engagement over the entire range of motion—not just certain parts of the exercise. The result: a stronger, fitter, and more energized body for your workout and beyond.

Choose the Right Dumbbells

While the size of weights that will challenge your muscles is very individual, it's ideal to have several different sizes to work with, even when you're starting out, because some muscles (like those in your lower body) are much stronger thanks to their daily job of carrying the rest of you around, whereas others (like in your upper body) tend to be a bit wimpier because they simply don't get worked as hard in everyday life.

Even within your arms there are differences: Your biceps, or the muscle in the front of your arm that flexes when you bend at the elbow (picture the classic "check out my muscle" pose), is stronger than the triceps, or the back of your arm that you use when you straighten your arm from a bent position. Trying to use the same weight for all the exercises is a bit like throwing a third grader into an eighth-grade classroom, or vice versa. You'll end up overwhelming your less-developed muscles and boring the stronger ones.

I recommend starting with, at the minimum, one set of smaller weights (3 or 5 pounds) and one set of larger weights (8 or 10 pounds). If you have even more options (such as a 3-, 5-, and 10-pounder), even better. Here's a quick guide to which exercises you're likely to be able to go heavy on, and which you'll be more successful starting with a smaller-size weight.

EXERCISE	MUSCLES WORKED	SUGGESTED WEIGHT
Two-Way Row	Arms and shoulders	Medium
Pickup and Shrug	Lower back, butt, back of thighs, shoulders	Heavy
Chest Press	Arms, chest	Medium to heavy
Side Leg-Lift Crunch	Hips, butt, obliques	Medium
Cheerleader Press	Shoulders, arms, triceps	Light to medium
Skater Side Twist	Hips, thighs, butt, obliques	Heavy (single dumbbell)
Pullover and Crunch	Triceps, abs	Light to medium
Lunge Repeater	Butt, hips, thighs, legs, arms	Medium
Butt Kicker	Butt, backs of thighs, abs	Medium
Squat and Curl	Butt, thighs, arms	Medium

Find Your Level

Working out at a level that feels good to you is the first step to seeing the results this program is designed to deliver. If you push yourself so hard that you end up too sore—or worse, injured—to stick with the plan, you'll hardly get where you're aiming to go. And similarly, if you continue to go through the motions of a routine that isn't challenging you, you won't find yourself getting much fitter that way either. Luckily, there are plenty of ways to adapt this program to fit your body and your life.

Frequency: We recommend doing two or three strength workouts a week during this program. While squeezing in three workouts will give you a slight advantage, don't feel guilty if you can only manage two. In fact, it turns out that those two workouts will give you roughly 90 percent of the benefits you'd see if you did three, so there are some serious diminishing returns going on. When Wayne Westcott, PhD, fitness research director at South Shore YMCA in Quincy, Massachusetts, and his colleagues reviewed data they'd collected on more than 1,600 exercisers across 8 years, they found that exercisers who strength trained twice a week gained exactly the same amount of lean muscle as those who strength trained three times a week. The thrice-weekly crew did have one thing to show for their time, though: They lost roughly 1 extra pound of body fat in 10 weeks—a nice bonus, but not so much you need to get down on yourself if a third workout isn't in the cards.

Sets and reps: Aim to do at least one set of 8 to 12 reps of each exercise each time you do the strength workout. When you start out, this might take you as much as 30 minutes to do, but once you get the hang of things, you should be able to do two sets in half an hour. Three sets will likely take you longer, so that's optional—it's better to do one or two if that's what you have time for than none! Quality trumps quantity in this program. It's better to do one or two sets of just 8 or 10 repetitions that leave your muscles spent than three sets of 12 reps that you finish feeling like you could do it all again. Researchers have long argued the pros and cons of lifting heavy weights just a few times versus light ones many times, but the most recent research suggests that when it comes to building muscle—the metabolism-boosting stuff we're after here—what really matters is that you finish each exercise feeling like you couldn't do another rep.

Resistance: You should be feeling stronger by now than you were when you started this program. In fact, by Week 3 of our test panel, subjects improved their upper-body strength by as much as 14 percent and their leg strength by twice that, 28 percent. But simply adding a dumbbell to the band you've been using may still be too much (especially if you've already bumped up the resistance of your band, which we hope you did in response to your newfound strength!). Don't be afraid to backtrack to a lighter resistance band, or use a smaller dumbbell to start. From there, you can follow a stair-stepping pattern to increase the resistance as needed, increasing the dumb-

REST FOR SUCCESS

How much to rest between exercise sets is a question that's regularly debated among exercise researchers and trainers alike. Like so many workout variables, the answer is "it depends." A competitive lifter whose goal is to lift the heaviest possible weight during each set might take as much as 5 minutes between sets to make sure his muscles are thoroughly rested before he attempts another set or the next exercise. Meanwhile, a different approach, often called circuit training, boasts big calorie burn and a bonus cardio element as a result of doing exercises back-to-back.

This workout will be most successful if you find a middle ground between those two approaches. After all, you do want to build that calorie-burning muscle we've been talking about, so you want your muscles to be rested enough to give each exercise your all. But who among us has the time to sit around for 5 minutes between sets?

In order to rest between sets without wasting time, I like to alternate upper-body and lower-body exercises as much as possible. That way, if you start with an arm move, then go on to a leg move, your arms will get a breather while your legs do the work. Another easy back-to-back technique: alternating arms or legs. When you do an exercise separately on two sides, no rest is needed. Unfortunately, one time-saving measure you'll see in some of the exercises in this book makes those techniques tricky. For exercises like the Squat and Curl, which use both upper and lower body and use both arms and legs concurrently, feel free to rest for a minute or so before going on to the next move.

bell, then the band. Just make sure your increases don't land you with a band you can't quite stretch through the full range of motion, warns Greg Niederlander, band expert with Spri, a fitness equipment company that provided some of the bands our test panelists used. If you get to that point, your resistance is too heavily weighted (bad pun!) toward the bands and you should decrease the band and add a heavier weight if you want to step it up.

Triple-Duty Toning Exercises

Do the exercises that follow just like you did during the first 3 weeks of the program. In the first week, it's okay if you need to drop back down to one or two sets of 8 to 12 repetitions, doing the routine twice over the course of the week. Once you get comfortable with the moves, work on increasing to two or three sets per workout, up to three times a week.

Looking for more of a challenge? You can always increase the resistance to up your effort. Or try the "Make It Harder" variations of each move, which introduce tweaks such as doing the exercise while balancing on one foot to help to work the muscles more (and in many cases, work extra stability muscles, like your core). If there's no "Make It Harder" exercise offered (or even if there is), remember that you can always make it harder by increasing the resistance of the bands, the dumbbells, or both.

If you find that one of the exercises in this chapter is too challenging, feel free to go back to the band-only version from the last chapter, or try the "Make It Easier" versions in Chapter 3 while adding the dumbbell.

Triple-Duty Two-Way Row

(feel it in your: arms and shoulders)

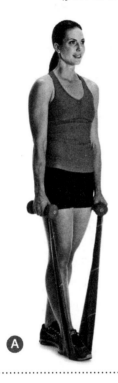

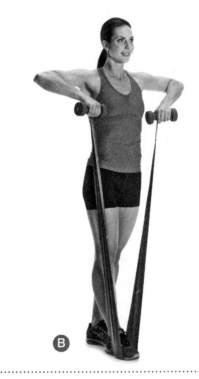

Step 1. Stand with your feet staggered, right foot forward with the middle of the band secured underfoot, one end in each hand along with a dumbbell, arms hanging at your sides (Photo A).

Step 2. With your palms facing back, bend your elbows out to the sides, stretching the band and lifting the dumbbells until they're at about chest height (Photo B).

Step 3. Pause; slowly lower to the starting position.

Step 4. Repeat the row, this time turning your wrists so your palms face in and your elbows point back as you pull up (Photo C). Continue alternating directions for 8 to 12 total reps per set (each pull counts as 1 rep). Switch the forward foot after each set.

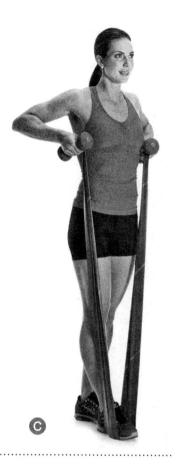

(C)

➡ *Faster Toning Tip*

Make sure to keep your shoulders down so they don't inch their way up toward your ears, creating tension in your neck. When you lift with your palms facing your sides and your elbows pointing back, imagine your shoulder blades drawing toward each other.

➡ *Make It Harder*

Balance on one leg as you do the move, band under the standing foot. Switch the balancing leg after each set (Photo D).

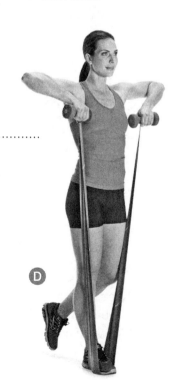

(D)

Triple-Duty Pickup and Shrug

(feel it in your: lower back, butt, and back of thighs)

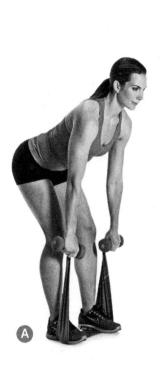

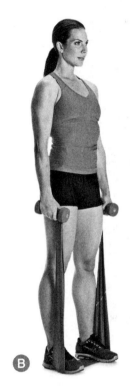

Step 1. Stand with your feet hip-width apart, the band centered under both feet, loose ends gripped in each hand along with a dumbbell.

Step 2. Keeping your abs tight to support your back, hinge from your hips to fold forward until your back is nearly parallel with the floor (Photo A).

Step 3. Choke up on the band so it's taut (try rotating your wrists so the band wraps around your hands and the dumbbells), then squeeze your glutes to lift your torso back to standing (Photo B).

Step 4. Shrug your shoulders toward your ears (Photo C). Repeat for 8 to 12 reps to complete 1 set.

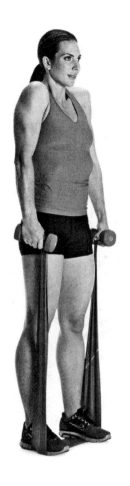

C

⟹ _Faster Toning Tip_

Focus on your posture with this move. Imagine there's a broomstick strapped to your back to keep it stable throughout the move. Keep your chest lifted, shoulder blades pulled back, and make sure not to round your back.

⟹ _Make It Harder_

Do the move balancing on one leg, band under the standing foot. Switch the balancing leg halfway through the set (Photo D).

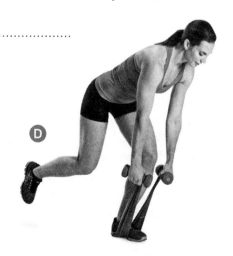

D

③

Triple-Duty Chest Press

(feel it in your: chest and arms)

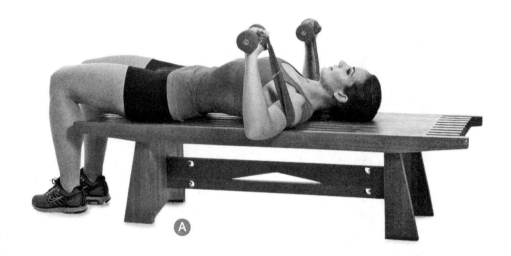

Ⓐ

Step 1. Lie on your back on a bench if you have one (a coffee table also works) or on the floor if you don't. Bend your knees to place your feet flat on the floor, band positioned under your upper back. Hold one end of the band plus a dumbbell in each hand, elbows bent and hands near your chest (Photo A).

Step 2. Press the weights and stretch the band straight up toward the ceiling until your arms are straight, but do not lock your elbows (Photo B).

Step 3. Pause, then slowly return to the starting position. Repeat for 8 to 12 reps to complete 1 set.

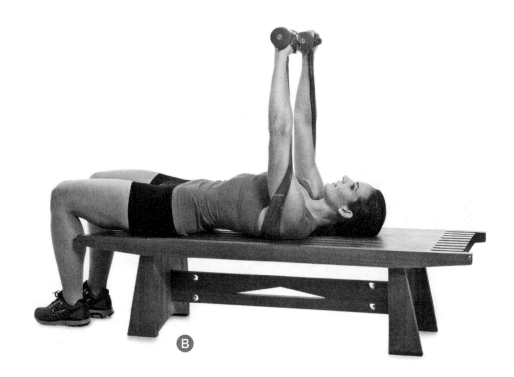

B

➡ *Faster Toning Tip*

Keep your shoulders down and away from your ears.

➡ *Make It Harder*

Lift your feet from the floor, knees bent 90 degrees and shins parallel to the floor (Photo C).

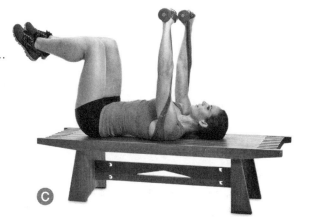

C

Triple-Duty Side Leg-Lift Crunch

(feel it in your: hips, butt, and obliques)

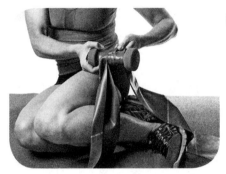

A

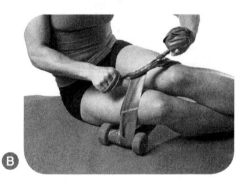

B

Step 1. Wrap the band several times around the middle of the dumbbell (Photo A), then securely tie the remainder of the band around your upper legs at arm's length (Photo B).

Step 2. Lie on your right side, legs stacked, right arm extended, and left hand on hip.

Step 3. Position the dumbbell to rest on the top of your legs (Photo C).

Step 4. Simultaneously raise your top leg while crunching your torso up (Photo D).

Step 5. Pause, then lower your torso and leg to the starting position. Repeat for 8 to 12 reps, then switch sides to complete 1 set.

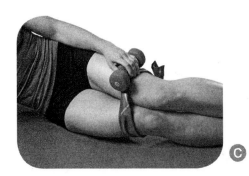

C

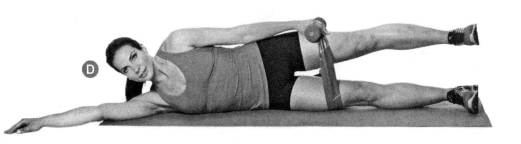

D

➡ Make It Harder

Don't lower your leg completely between reps; raise and lower it without touching the lower leg.

➡ Faster Toning Tip

Imagine your body is sandwiched between two panes of glass. Try to keep your body in a straight line as you lift your torso and your leg so you don't touch the glass.

5

Triple-Duty Cheerleader Press

(feel it in your: shoulders, arms, and triceps)

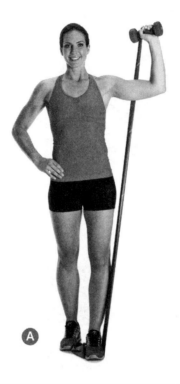

Ⓐ

Step 1. Stand with your feet slightly staggered, left forward, one end of the band under your left foot with the free end plus a dumbbell gripped in your left hand. Wrap the band around your hand if you have extra length.

Step 2. Bend your left elbow about 90 degrees and raise your arm until your upper arm is at chest level, palm facing forward (Photo A).

Step 3. Press straight up overhead (Photo B). That's 1 rep.

Step 4. Bend your elbow to lower your forearm behind you (Photo C) and press up again. That's 2 reps. Do 8 to 12 reps, then switch sides to complete a set.

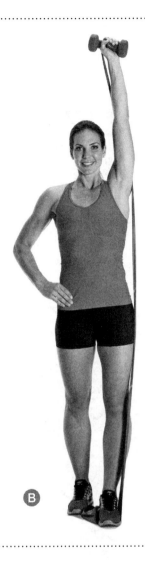

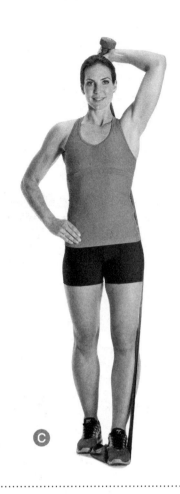

➡ *Faster Toning Tip*

To get the most upper-arm firming out of this move, try to keep your upper arm still as your forearm bends behind you and then presses back up.

Triple-Duty Skater Side Twist

(feel it in your: hips, thighs, butt, and obliques)

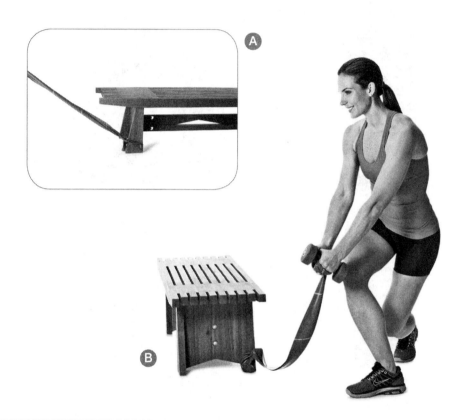

Step 1. Tie the band to a low, sturdy object like the leg of a piece of heavy furniture (Photo A).

Step 2. Standing with the anchored band to your right, grasp both ends of the band and a single dumbbell together in both hands.

Step 3. Step diagonally back and to the right with your left foot, and bend both knees about 45 degrees as though into a curtsy (Photo B).

Step 4. Stand, toes pointing forward, then rotate your torso toward the right side (Photo C). Repeat for 8 to 12 reps, then switch sides to complete a set.

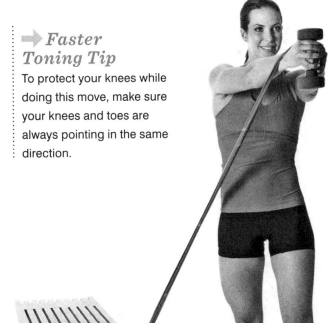

➡ *Faster Toning Tip*

To protect your knees while doing this move, make sure your knees and toes are always pointing in the same direction.

Ⓒ

➡ *Make It Harder*

Add a balance challenge by reaching your left foot back without touching as you bend your right knee about 45 degrees into a single-leg squat (Photo D).

Ⓓ

Triple-Duty Pullover and Crunch

(feel it in your: triceps and abs)

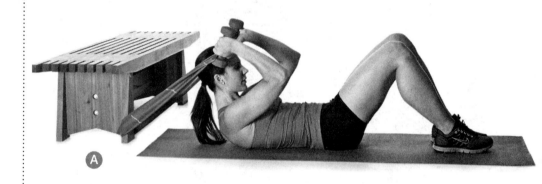

Step 1. Loop the band around a sturdy object like the leg of a piece of heavy furniture. Lie on your back with your head in front of the anchored band, knees bent, and feet flat on the floor.

Step 2. Bending your elbows, reach back to grasp one end of the band, along with a dumbbell, in each hand, arms bent about 90 degrees and elbows near your ears.

Step 3. Engage your abs to crunch upward (Photo A).

Step 4. Press the weights forward, straightening, but not locking, your elbows (Photo B).

Step 5. Slowly lower your body, then your arms. Do 8 to 12 reps to complete a set.

➡ *Faster Toning Tip*

To maximize firming in the backs of your upper arms (aka the chicken wings), try to keep your upper arms stationary as you straighten your elbows forward.

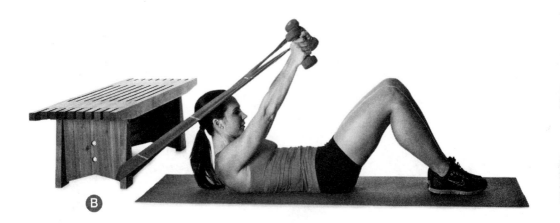

B

➡ *Make It Harder*

Lift your feet off the floor as you do the move, bending your knees to 90 degrees with your shins parallel to the floor (Photo C). To enhance, point your toes.

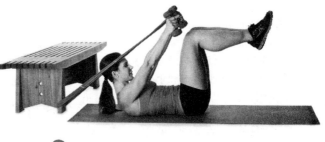

C

8

Triple-Duty Lunge Repeater

(feel it in your: butt, hips, thighs, and legs)

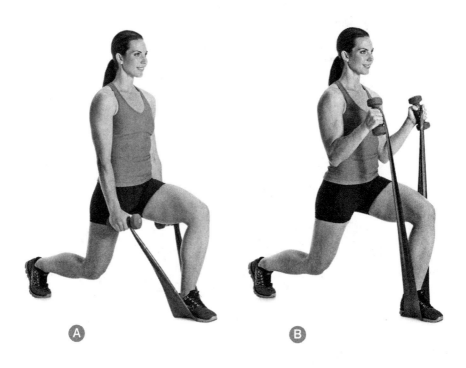

Step 1. Stand with your feet hip-width apart, the center of the band under your left foot. Hold one end of the band and a dumbbell in each hand, arms at sides, palms facing in.

Step 2. Take a big step backward with your right foot, bending both knees to lower into a lunge with your left knee over your ankle (Photo A).

Step 3. Bend your elbows and curl your hands toward your shoulders, rotating your arms so your palms face your chest (Photo B).

Step 4. Step forward to stand (Photo C). Slowly lower your arms. Do 8 to 12 reps per side to complete a set.

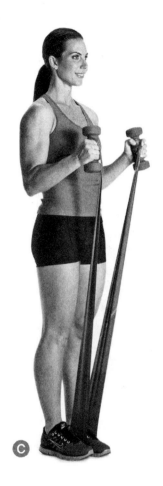

➡ *Faster Toning Tip*

Timing is key to getting the most out of this move. Make sure you keep your hands curled up toward your shoulders until you've returned to standing in order to maximize thigh and butt toning.

➡ *Make It Harder*

Don't touch your foot when you step your back foot forward out of the lunge (Photo D).

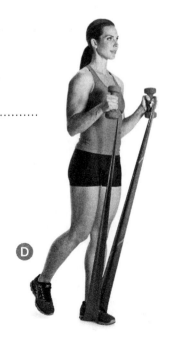

Triple-Duty Butt Kicker

(feel it in your: butt, backs of thighs, and abs)

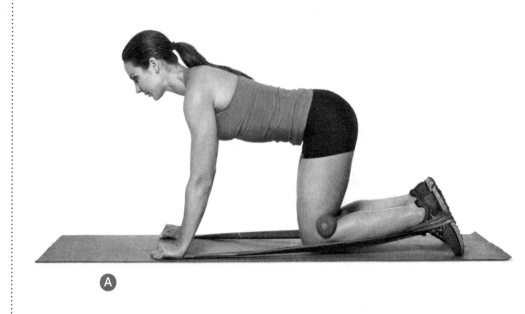

Ⓐ

Step 1. Get into a tabletop position on your hands and knees, wrists below shoulders and knees below hips.

Step 2. Wrap the band around your left heel and place a dumbbell behind your bent left knee. Grasp one end of the band in each hand (Photo A). (Tip: Crisscrossing the ends of the band and hooking the band underneath the two ends of the dumbbell helped some testers keep it all together.)

Step 3. Keeping your left foot flexed, press your left heel up and back, squeezing the dumbbell behind your knee (Photo B). Repeat 8 to 12 times, then switch legs and repeat to complete a set.

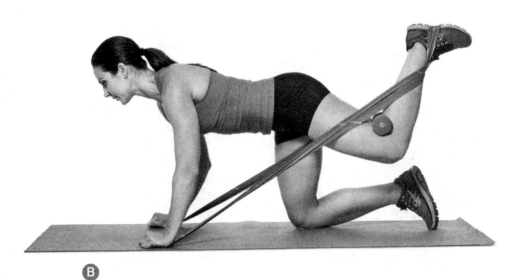

B

⇒ Make It Harder
Don't touch your knee down
between reps.

**⇒ Faster
Toning Tip**
To avoid neck or back
strain—and to get a bit of
bonus core strength from
this move—keep your neck
in line with your spine, your
back flat, and your abs
pulled up and in as you do
this exercise.

Triple-Duty Squat and Curl

(feel it in your: butt, thighs, and arms)

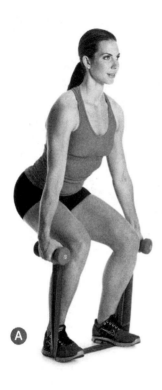

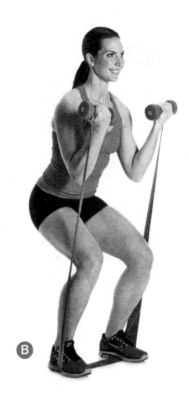

Step 1. Stand with your feet hip-width apart, a band under both feet, a loose end plus a dumbbell in each hand, palms facing your sides.

Step 2. Bend your knees to sit back, keeping your knees behind your toes (Photo A).

Step 3. Bend your elbows to curl your forearms upward (Photo B), rotating your wrists so your palms face your chest.

Step 4. Press into your heels to stand (Photo C), then slowly lower your arms back to the starting position. Do 8 to 12 reps to complete a set.

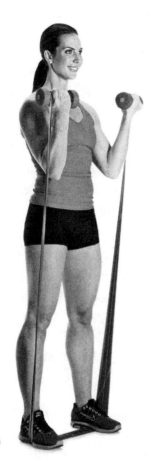

➡ Faster Toning Tip

Keep your upper arms glued to your sides as you curl your forearms up toward your shoulders, and make sure not to reverse the movement until you've risen out of the squat position.

C

➡ Make It Harder

Do a one-legged squat, bending your right knee and lifting your foot to the back as you bend your left knee and sit back to about 45 degrees (Photo D). Curl your arms up, then return to standing before lowering your arms.

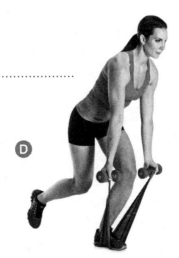

D

Common Questions about Dumbbells

Q It's hard enough to do the exercises with the band. How will I be able to lift a dumbbell, too?

A Many of our testers were ready to step up their resistance level at this point in the program, so they were able to add a dumbbell and continue to use the same band. However, if you're already using a challenging band (good for you!), it's okay to back off to a lighter resistance band in order to be able to complete a set with both band and dumbbell. Remember, it's all right if you can only do 8 reps to start—especially when you have just increased your resistance level. In fact, it's actually *better* to do 8 reps and not be able to do another without a rest than it is to do 12 and feel like you could keep going.

Q How do I determine the right combo of band and dumbbell resistance for me?

A In the original study from Ithaca College, the researchers used a fish scale to measure the elastic resistance in order to balance the weight so 20 percent of the challenge was coming from the band and 80 percent from the dumbbells. But you don't have to be that scientific about it. Just make sure you're getting a good amount of resistance from both tools, erring toward the dumbbell weight. In other words, if you're using a 1-pound weight and the heaviest band you have, I'd suggest you bump the weight up—even if you have to decrease the band's resistance. And if you're hoisting a 10-pounder along with the lightest resistance band, drop down the weight a bit if you need to in order to use a thicker band. Also, because weights can be found in intervals of as little as 2 or 3 pounds whereas bands are more limited (they typically come in extra light, light, medium, heavy, and extra or "special" heavy), you'll want to increase the size of the dumbbell more frequently.

To Gym or Not to Gym

The beauty of this plan is that it can be done anywhere—including your very own living room. If you don't like having to go anywhere for a workout (besides out the door for cardio), home is most probably where you'll stick with it. But if you're already a member at a gym or YMCA, there are plenty of reasons to go: unlimited equipment options, the energizing buzz of other exercisers, free towel service. Whichever routine you choose, here are a few do's and don'ts.

At the Gym

Don't fear the free weight area. In some gyms, free weights are sequestered off into a separate area from the weight machines. Even if there are men lifting giant weights, don't be intimidated—you belong there, too. (Don't worry, grunting isn't required.)

Do use the mirrors. It may seem like the ultimate in narcissism, but those mirrored walls are there for more than admiring yourself. Looking at your reflection as you do an exercise allows you to check up on your mechanics without screwing up your form by looking down.

Don't be afraid to ask the staff questions. You don't have to hire a personal trainer to get tips. If you're not sure if you're doing an exercise correctly, ask a trainer or group exercise instructor to take a look. Chances are he or she will be happy to help.

Do take advantage of lots of equipment options. Having an entire rack of different-size weights at your disposal means you can experiment with different sizes for different exercises without having to devote a room of your house to dumbbells. Don't hesitate to try a heavier weight—worst-case scenario is you put it back on the rack and go back to the smaller one. Use the bench, too, for your chest presses. While you can do this exercise on the floor, you'll get a better range of motion on a bench.

Don't forget to put the equipment back. Nobody likes a messy exerciser.

Do go with a friend. The more the merrier! (Just be sure she's not more into chatting than exercising. If she is, better to plan your sweat date for an easy cardio day.)

At Home

Do turn on some tunes. Research has found that listening to upbeat music improves your mood and makes exercise feel easier (or lets you work out harder without its feeling harder). Can't argue with that!

Don't watch TV. Okay, if it's the difference between skipping your workout in favor of watching the season finale of *Dancing with the Stars*

BEYOND THE DUMBBELL

While this book focuses on bands and dumbbells, there are many other tools that can help you to strengthen and tone your muscles. Here's a rundown of some of our favorites, along with the pros and cons of each.

Kettlebells

What they are: These traditionally solid-iron weights that look like a cannonball with a handle have been coated in colored vinyl for a less-intimidating appearance now that they've become popular with everyday exercisers. By holding the handle and swinging the weight as you do different movements, you engage the whole body in just about every move.

Why they're great: There are few indoor workouts that can so closely mimic the full-body heave-ho required to do something like shoveling snow from your driveway. Plus, the dynamic movements have been shown to burn up to 60 percent more calories than traditional weights.

What's not so great: Learning how to use kettlebells safely—and effectively—is best done with the help of a pro. After all, swinging around a weighted ball can do some serious shoulder damage if done improperly—let alone living room damage if you accidentally drop it or let go midswing.

Medicine Balls

What they are: Weighted rubber balls you can hold or throw.

Why they're great: Working out just seems more fun and gamelike when you add a ball. They are ideal for core exercises because you can

---

or doing your workout during the show, I'll compromise. But know that you'll get the best results from your strength workout if you focus on the exercise you're doing. Your mind is a more powerful part of your workout than you think. In fact, in a study from the Cleveland Clinic in Ohio, exercisers who just imagined flexing their biceps as hard as they could (electrical sensors hooked up to the testers' arms made sure they didn't

hold the ball as you do crunches and twists. You can also throw and catch with a partner, which uses your core for stabilization.

What's not so great: There are fewer exercises you can do with a medicine ball compared with a simple band or dumbbell.

Barbells

What they are: Found in many gyms, barbells are a metal rod onto which you can add different-size plates until you have the perfect amount of weight. Don't forget to add the weight of the bar to the weight of the plates or you might be lifting more than you think!

Why they're great: They give you much more extensive weight options without taking up the space of dozens of dumbbells.

What's not so great: You have to take them apart and put them back together every time you want to use a different weight.

Weight Machines

What they are: The bread and butter of most health clubs from Curves to the YMCA is a circuit-training room where you can go from machine to machine, do what's instructed, and be guaranteed a full-body workout.

Why they're great: Machines are fairly safe and foolproof and require little instruction to figure out.

What's not so great: Because the movement is controlled by the machine and typically focuses on isolating specific muscles, the exercises aren't as relatable to real-world movements.

actually flex) increased their strength by 13.5 percent. The "exercisers" came into the clinic five times a week for a 15-minute "training" program that involved performing "mental contractions" of the biceps, or the muscle that flexes the elbow. Researchers believe the gains were thanks to improved signaling between the brain and the muscle. Other studies have also demonstrated how important it is to tune in to your workout. In a study published in the *Journal of Strength and Conditioning Research,* Australian researchers demonstrated that exercisers who gave themselves a mini pep talk to psych themselves up before doing a strength-training exercise produced 18 percent more force than peers who were distracted before performing the move.

Do find a mirror if you can. Leave the heavy grunters behind, but using a mirror to watch your form is one trick worth stealing from the gym. If you have a full-length mirror in your bedroom or on the back of a door somewhere in your house with enough space for exercise, use it!

Keeping Track of Your Workouts

Just like with the band workout, knowing how many sets and reps you did last time and which bands and dumbbells to grab for each move can help you to make your workouts more efficient—and more effective. It's also a good reminder of when you might be ready to jump to the next size dumbbell or increase the resistance level of your band (for example, if you've been doing several sets of 12 reps for a few workouts in a row). And of course it still serves as a good checklist to make sure you don't forget any moves.

See a sample log at right. For a blank log page you can copy and use, flip to page 307 in the Tone Every Inch Logs.

Triple-Duty Toning Workout Log

Week of program: (5) **Date:** _4/1/12_

EXERCISE	REPS	WEIGHT USED (COLOR OF BAND AND/OR SIZE OF DUMBBELL)	OBSERVATIONS/ CHALLENGES
Triple-Duty Two-Way Row	10/10	Green band/5-lb weight	
Triple-Duty Pickup and Shrug	12/12	Blue band/5-lb weight	Increase weight next time.
Triple-Duty Chest Press	10/8	Blue band/5-lb weight	Barely finished the second set!
Triple-Duty Side Leg-Lift Crunch	12/10	Green band/5-lb weight	
Triple-Duty Cheerleader Press	8/8	Green band/3-lb weight	
Triple-Duty Skater Side Twist	12/12	Blue band/10-lb weight	
Triple-Duty Pullover and Crunch	10/8	Green band/5-lb weight	Tough one
Triple-Duty Lunge Repeater	12/10	Blue band/8-lb weight	
Triple-Duty Butt Kicker	12/12	Green band/5-lb weight	Try blue band next time.
Triple-Duty Squat and Curl	12/10	Blue band/5-lb weight	

Barbara Terrell
Age 54

Lost: 7 percent body fat

Gained: 32 percent stronger legs and 25 percent stronger arms

Favorite sculpted body part: Her whittled waistline

Favorite on-the-go meal: Greek yogurt with cereal

Barb Terrell was the strength-training veteran of the Tone Every Inch test panel. "I love lifting heavy weights," she says. Unfortunately, the heavy weights didn't love her body back, because using them often forced her to sacrifice good form, lose flexibility, and aggravate her chronic shoulder pain. So despite an already fairly regimented routine of free weights and cardio, Barb decided to give this new program a shot.

Initially she was a skeptic. "With the bands, at first I was like, 'Oh brother, I'm not doing very much here,'" she says. "But then I realized how much the bands were also working other stabilizing muscles—like your core—that you don't even realize they're working." One of the best stealth moves that helped to firm and narrow her waist more than anything she'd tried in the past: the

Skater Side Twist. "It's really a tiny move, so I was surprised at the impact that it had on me," she says.

The back was another trouble area for Barb, for which the bands proved a good remedy. "I can wear certain tops now without back overhang from my bra," she says. The bands also helped Barb to feel stronger without sacrificing the range of motion always lost when she used free weights by themselves. "The bands give me a wider range of motion, cover more muscles in just a couple of exercises, and help keep me flexible."

And as important as she believes weights are, it's the Intensity Cardio that Barb credits with keeping her belly fat down. "I'd say my stomach is firmer since I started doing intervals," she says. A dedicated exerciser from the start, she found that pairing the band workouts with cardio on the same day provided the most improvement. "I liked the way my body responded to that," she says. "My arms have more definition, my pants fit looser, and I can't pinch as much excess in the waist area anymore."

While she didn't follow the diet religiously, Barb became more aware of her eating habits and did make an effort to eat more protein—something she knew she wasn't getting enough of—as well as more fresh produce. Because she wasn't much of a meat-eater, Greek yogurt became a go-to protein source that helped to keep her feeling full longer, whether she ate it first thing in the morning stirred into oatmeal or mixed with bran cereal, or had a 4-ounce single-serve cup as an afternoon snack. "I try not to make changes I don't think I can keep up for a lifetime since I don't want to set myself up for failure," Barb says, explaining her aversion to so-called diets. "Yet it's interesting how despite not making any huge changes, I could make this obvious change in my body composition," she says of her 7 percent reduction in body fat. "At almost 55, I try to be thankful I can hold my own!"

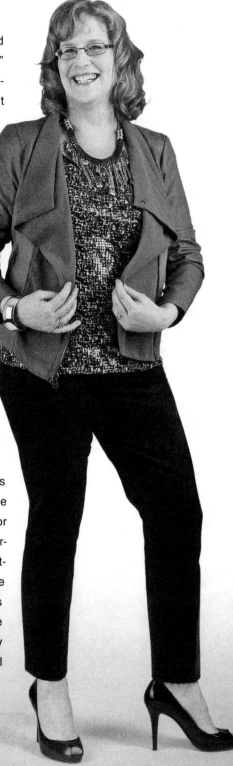

Kick It Up with Cardio

Although strength comes first in this program, it's still important not to leave out the cardio, for a few reasons. Aerobic exercise comes with its own set of benefits for all-around health and weight loss that make a great complement to resistance training.

Studies have found that a dose of brisk walking can lower your risk of heart disease, stroke, diabetes, certain types of cancer, and depression. And because it's best to work on toning no more than two or three times a week in order to give those muscles a chance to recover and adapt to the stress of strengthening, adding cardio offers an opportunity to squeeze in some energizing feel-good exercise on the in-between days.

Why Cardio?

Getting your heart pumping is good for more than burning calories (and helping you break a sweat). Test panelist Barbara Terrell swears by the power of pairing sculpting exercises with cardio (especially belly-firming intervals). "I love the energy it gives me," she says, "and I am a firm believer that interval cardio helps with belly fat." Here are just a few of my favorite reasons to lace up those running (or walking) shoes.

Beef Up Brainpower

Numerous studies have shown that aerobic exercise helps to maintain and even improve your brain health, thanks in part to increased blood-flow and glucose to the brain. And while a few studies have suggested positive effects from strength training, cardio is leading the charge in this area. As you get older, staying aerobically active may protect your memory by slowing or even reversing age-related brain shrinkage linked to dementia and Alzheimer's disease. In a study of 120 older adults, who would typically be expected to experience shrinking of the hippocampus at their ages (the hippocampus is a part of the brain that controls memory), those who walked on a track actually *increased* the size of the hippocampal region of the brain by 2 percent (compared with the 1.4 percent reduction experienced by the nonwalking control group). That's equivalent to turning back the clock a year or two, explain the authors in the journal *Proceedings of the National Academy of Sciences*.

Short bursts of intense cardio (like the interval workouts described later in this chapter) could help you buff up your vocab too. Exercisers who ran hard for 3 minutes, then rested for 2, then repeated the sequence, learned new words 20 percent faster than those who just relaxed before their lesson, found German researchers from the University of Muenster. Maybe it's time to learn a new language.

Ease Hormone Woes

Chill out, hot flashes. Canadian researchers discovered that brisk walking was just what the doctor ordered for leveling out the weight gain and headaches some women experience in conjunction with the hormonal shifts of menopause. Aerobically active women in the study, who ranged from age 39 to 82, had 44 percent fewer headaches and were 22 percent less likely to report weight gain compared with more sedentary counterparts.

Meanwhile, German researchers found that a combo of weights and walking relieved hot flashes and night sweats as well as hormone therapy (and with a lot fewer side effects!). For women who haven't hit that stage yet, studies also suggest that regular aerobic activity can improve symptoms of PMS.

Help Beat Diabetes

Cardio is one of your best defenses against type 2 diabetes, the kind that typically sets in later in life and is attributed largely to lifestyle factors. In fact, daily walking was shown to be capable of reversing early symptoms of diabetes—improving insulin sensitivity as well as the ability to produce insulin, both of which demonstrate better blood sugar control—in as little as 7 days, according to a University of Michigan study.

And combining strength and cardio exercise has been shown to offer more benefits than either type of training provides on its own. In research led by Timothy S. Church at the Pennington Biomedical Research Center in Baton Rouge, Louisiana, scientists assigned diabetic men and women ranging from their forties to their sixties to either an aerobic exercise, strength exercise, or combined routine, all requiring roughly the same time commitment for exercise. Only the group that combined cardio and resistance training improved their levels of a type of hemoglobin in the blood that is a measurement of blood sugar control. As a bonus, the group that took a two-pronged approach also lost nearly twice as much weight during the 9-month trial.

Amp Up the Intensity

Not all cardio is created equal. The cornerstone of the cardio in this plan is all about adding intensity. If you already do some cardio, but the scale isn't budging, intensity may be the missing ingredient. For most of us, if we go out for a walk, or even for a run, our bodies naturally find their most efficient pace. Well, let me tell you, efficiency is good for a lot of things—getting work done, cleaning the house, even finishing your workout—but while you're exercising, the last thing you want is for your body to be too efficient. That's because efficiency for your body means conserving calories and fat—hardly the goal if you're trying to lose weight!

Slow and Steady Doesn't Burn Much Fat

If you've ever watched a marathon, you might have been surprised to see the number of overweight runners and walkers crossing the finish line. After all, shouldn't all the miles of training they logged to traverse a rigorous 26.2 miles have left them looking like beanpoles? Now don't get me wrong . . . finishing a marathon is a great feat whatever your weight, and there are plenty of reasons to do it that have nothing to do with weight loss. Moreover, signing up for a road race, whether it's a 5-K, a marathon, or something in between, can be a great motivator both throughout the training and on the day of the race. I've run one marathon myself, walked a half-marathon with my mom and a group of *Prevention* magazine readers, and cheered from the sidelines for countless others. I'll be the first to say that there's nothing more inspirational than standing on a starting line before dawn with a crowd of men and women, nerves jangling, numbers pinned on T-shirts, excitedly awaiting the starting gun.

But just like we talked about in the last chapter with the strength workout, this program is about quality, not quantity. Not only do you not have to walk or run for an hour or more a day to lose weight and inches (in fact, marathoners commonly go out for several hours or more for their training!), you can actually achieve *better* results in *less* time. Yes, really! You can see the potential for time savings by looking at the government's physical activity guidelines, which recommend $2\frac{1}{2}$ hours a week (for example, 30 minutes, five times weekly) if you're doing moderate intensity. Kick it up to high intensity and you only have to do $1\frac{1}{4}$ hours weekly. In other words, just by pumping up the intensity, you can cut the duration of your workouts in half while still meeting the government's exercise goals, according to the Centers for Disease Control and Prevention.

The Shortcut That Takes Off Six Times the Weight

Take two workouts: One involves 40 minutes of biking, the other just 20 minutes. Which workout do you think would yield more weight loss? Australian researchers did just that test with two groups of women. To level the playing field, they added a twist: Despite the different workout durations, both groups of women pedaled off the same number of calories (about 200) using stationary bikes.

How is that possible? The 20-minute group had to pick up the intensity in order to burn more calories in less time, so they alternated short 8-second sprints with slightly longer 12-second recovery bouts of slow pedaling. The 40-minute group of women biked at a steady pace for twice as long. You might be thinking that identical calories burned means they must have lost the same amount of weight. And that alone would be a fairly impressive finding—that you can lose the same amount of weight in half the time just by adding some short sprints.

But the real findings were even more impressive than that. The speedsters didn't just match the weight lost by their peers, they exceeded it by six times. The numbers weren't huge (3 pounds for the sprint group versus ½ pound for the steady cyclists), but they're all the more impressive given the fact that the women in the study were in their twenties and already pretty lean at the start.

But the benefits aren't just for the young and already fit. In another study, this one conducted here in the United States at the University of Virginia in Charlottesville, researchers had two groups of overweight, middle-aged women start walking far enough to burn 400 calories a day, 5 days a week. One group walked at a steady moderate pace (slightly faster than 18 minutes per mile), whereas the second group walked the same 5 days, but on 3 of the days they pushed the pace to about 16 minutes per mile. So they walked off the exact same number of calories but at slightly different walking speeds. How do you think the results stacked up?

Well, the power walkers won again. They lost 66 percent more total weight, including more than twice as much pure fat. One possible explanation is that maintaining speedier paces requires more muscle power, which may help to preserve lean muscle tissue. That means weight loss is focused on fat, not muscle, which you know by now is über-important to keeping your metabolism buzzing along briskly. Of that fat, the high-intensity group lost more than three times as much subcutaneous fat (the kind you can pinch) and more than twice as much dangerous visceral fat (the kind that surrounds the organs and increases your disease risk). And perhaps most impressively, they lost an amazing five times the abdominal fat as the slowgoers did. All from shaving just a couple minutes per mile off their walking pace!

Add Intensity with Intervals

One of the most popular ways to add intensity is with a technique called intervals—the technical term for what the Australian exercisers did in the first study I talked about earlier. The gist: You push yourself harder than you normally would for a brief period, then slow down to catch your breath (and let your muscles at least partially refuel their energy stores) before you go again.

Interval workouts are more challenging than steady-paced moderate workouts, but they give you a lot more bang for your buck. And they work fast. Studies have shown that picking up the intensity for short spurts may improve your fitness (meaning your heart and lungs' ability to pump oxygen and fuel your muscles) in as little as 2 weeks. You could get similar benefits with long, slow endurance training—it would just take you a heck of a lot longer. And improved fitness isn't just good for competitive athletes. It means you feel more energized doing your workouts and in your everyday life, so you're less likely to feel winded carrying groceries in from the car or rushing up a set of stairs.

Another benefit you'll see in as little as 2 weeks: a jump start to your body's fat-burning engines. In one study led by Martin Gibala, PhD, chair of the department of kinesiology at McMaster University in Hamilton, Ontario, who specializes in studying the metabolic changes spurred by interval workouts, researchers found that doing interval training increased the body's capacity to spin stored fat into usable energy by 36 percent in just 14 days. That boost is at least in part due to an increase in the number of mitochondria (the fancy term for powerhouses in your muscles that use oxygen to burn calories). In fact, Dr. Gibala's most recent research reveals that this increase in mitochondria action happens after a single interval workout. How's that for instant gratification!

Give Yourself a Break

All these arguments for high-intensity workouts don't mean that moderate cardio is worthless. After all, pushing your body hard all the time can lead to burnout and injuries. And the same way you need to take a day between strength-training workouts to allow your muscles to repair themselves and reap the benefits of their improved strength and tone, you need to give your body a break between vigorous cardio workouts to recover as well. That's why we never recommend doing more than three intensity workouts in a week, even in the final weeks of the program.

Besides, taking it easier has its own benefits, too. In fact, researchers at Duke University in Durham, North Carolina, found moderate cardio to be better than more vigorous workouts at controlling triglycerides, a type of fat in the bloodstream that increases your risk of heart disease. Studies have also shown that even short bouts of moderate cardio (think: a short 15-minute walk around the block) can almost instantly boost energy levels, decrease depression, and even quell chocolate cravings.

So we have moderate-intensity exercise on this plan to balance out the tougher Intensity Cardio and toning workouts you'll be doing. In the first week of the plan, when everything is new, you'll stick to Moderate Cardio to get your heart pumping and loosen up tight muscles since you might be feeling extra sore from the strength routine.

You can do virtually any activity you like for these Moderate Cardio workouts, so feel free to get creative. Pop in a cardio dance DVD or go out dancing with your husband; head out into the great outdoors to go

GET YOUR SPOUSE IN ON THE ACTION

Want to know the secret of regular exercisers? They're three times more likely to have a spouse who's active as well, according to a University of Pittsburgh study. Whether you recruit your husband to join you on this plan (several of the women in our test panel did), or he prefers to do his own thing, a mutual understanding of the importance of fitting in your workouts will help to keep you both on track. *Prevention* magazine fitness columnist Chris Freytag swears by weekend runs with her hubby to catch up on their respective busy weeks, make parenting decisions, and log some quality together time. Plus, it's likely to boost your fitness *and* your love life thanks to those mood-boosting endorphins, enhanced bloodflow to the genitals, and perked-up body confidence.

→ **Helpful Hints:** Head Here to Find Workout Pals

Cheaper than a personal trainer (and arguably a lot more fun), pairing up with a workout buddy is a great way to maximize results. For one thing, planning to meet up for workouts keeps you accountable— you're more likely to feel guilty about standing up a friend than you are standing up yourself. But working out à deux also makes it *feel* easier, even as you push yourself to the max! In a study from the University of Oxford in England, rowers got twice the endorphin high (measured by how much discomfort they could withstand) when they did a tough workout in sync with their teammates as they did when performing the same effort solo. If you don't have exercise partners on speed dial, here are some good resources to get you started.

Prevention.com. Post on the Walking section of *Prevention* magazine's discussion boards to find other walkers near you who are looking for company.

Meetup.com. Surf over to this Web site and create a free profile in order to find or start a group that meets to do any activity you could use some company for: walking, running, hiking, or even ballroom dancing!

RRCA.org. The Road Runners Club of America is the largest conglomeration of running clubs in the country, and their Web site allows you to search for clubs near you. Don't worry about being fast enough. Most clubs include members who run (or even walk) at a variety of paces, so you're sure to find someone your speed. You can also find groups via bulletin boards at gyms, YMCAs, and community centers.

Sign up for a 5-K. Ready to get your competitive juices flowing? Road races often raise money for great causes, from cancer research to local schools, and they're a great place to meet prospective exercise buddies. Think of it as a healthier version of picking up a date at a bar—except it's the runner's high rather than beer putting people in extra-friendly moods.

hiking or walk around the neighborhood with a friend; go swimming or try a water aerobics class. Make these sessions an exercise in seeking out fun ways to move your body. While cardio machines at the gym are certainly an option, they're not the only way. Instead of striding away aimlessly on a treadmill watching reruns of bad TV shows, find (or form) a walking group in your community. Ingraining exercise into your social life is one of the best secrets of fit folks.

In the second week (Phase I), you'll swap out one Moderate Cardio workout for an Intensity Cardio workout, and you'll gradually increase that as you get fitter and stronger, until in the final weeks of the program your only required cardio will be the Intensity workouts. But perhaps you'll have a standing date to go hiking on Saturday mornings by then, and there's no need to skip it. Just think of it as extra credit.

A la Carte Cardio

Aerobic exercise is hardly one-size-fits-all. Some folks love biking, while others would rather get around on their own two feet. Some like the scenery of outdoor workouts, while others thrive on the buzz of a packed gym surrounded by other exercisers. That's why this plan is all about choice. You can choose any type of exercise that you like to do: walking, running, biking, swimming, using cardio machines; the options go on and on—kind of like the menu at your favorite Chinese restaurant.

Simply pick your exercise modality, and depending on what week of the program you're on, choose from the menu that fits: Moderate or Intensity. The easiest way to measure the intensity of your workout is by using the rate of perceived exertion (RPE), a scale of how you feel during your workout. For Moderate, you do your chosen workout at a steady effort of about a 5 or 6 (see "Quick Guide to RPE" for an explanation of the levels). For Intensity, you can choose from the five workout options starting on page 109. And unlike choosing a gym or a cell phone plan, there's no commitment! Just because you biked your workout on Monday doesn't mean you can't walk on Thursday. And if you chose the Fat Blast 30-Second Intervals for your last Intensity Cardio workout, you're

QUICK GUIDE TO RPE

Each of the workouts that follow is based on an effort scale of 1 to 10, where 1 is you sitting on the couch, and 10 is you sprinting for your life. Here's a quick reference guide to everything in between.

LEVEL	WHAT IT FEELS LIKE
1	Sitting on the couch
2–3	Standing, maybe strolling leisurely
4–5	Walking purposefully
6–7	Walking like you're late for a meeting
8–9	Chasing a bus that's about to pull away
10	Sprinting as fast as you can—even if you can only keep it up for 10 seconds or less

welcome to do it again or try out the Ab Blast Shortcut 8-Second Intervals this time. It's all about sampling the options to figure out what you like (or what you're in the mood for today). See "Your Choice Cardio" on page 114 for some tips on trying different types of cardio workouts.

Menu 1: Moderate Cardio

Choose from any of the workouts that follow to log the recommended amount of moderate cardio time each week, aiming for an effort level of about a 5 or 6 (see "Quick Guide to RPE"). For these types of workouts, there's no need to do a separate warmup or cooldown. You can build it right into your workout, by starting at a slower pace and picking it up as you feel warm and your muscles loosen up. At the end of the workout, you can gradually slow the pace for the last couple of minutes if stopping suddenly feels too abrupt (otherwise, your walk to the shower or wherever you're headed next is a perfectly adequate cooldown for a moderate intensity session). If you have time, postworkout is ideal to throw in a few minutes of stretching. See the stretching routine on page 180 for a full-body flexibility session.

You'll start with as little as 20 minutes of Moderate Cardio in Week 1 and increase it to 30 minutes per workout after that (longer if you feel like it). But don't despair if you can't hit those numbers. Do what you can—even if it's just 15 minutes one day. You can also split up these workouts over the course of the day, piecing together chunks of as little as 5 minutes at a time (a couple laps of the soccer field while you're waiting for your child to wrap up with practice, for example).

If you enjoy playing a sport like tennis or basketball, that counts, too, as long as it involves more moving than standing around. You can do more than 30 minutes a day if you like—perhaps taking an hour-long cardio class at the gym, or going for a long weekend walk with a friend. Here are some examples to get you started, but remember this list is just the beginning. If you want to add an activity not listed here, just make sure it's not a muscle-building workout (no weights, no resistance bands), and keep your exertion to a medium level—heart pumping, but no gasping for breath.

MODERATE CARDIO OPTIONS	CALORIES BURNED PER 30 MINUTES*
Cardio exercise DVD	Varies
Jogging	238–340
Swimming	238–340
Stair machine	300
Step aerobics	289
Outdoor cycling	272
Elliptical machine	238
Rowing machine	238
Stationary bike	238
Cardio dance class	221
Hiking	204
Mowing the lawn with a push mower	204
Ballroom dancing	100–187
Walking	112–170
Dancing around your house	153
Washing the car by hand	153
Water aerobics	136

*Based on a 150-pound exerciser. If you weigh more, your number will be higher. If you weigh less, your number will be lower.

Menu 2: Intensity Cardio

For each of the workouts that follow, choose your exercise modality (such as walking, running, biking, swimming, or anything you can adjust the intensity of according to the workout). Then simply follow the instructions. See page 114 for tips on different workouts you might want to try.

If you're short on time, feel free to skimp on the cooldown (you can cool down your body just as effectively en route to the shower as you can on the treadmill), but make sure to warm up adequately. Getting your muscles loose before you try to push yourself to go fast has myriad benefits: It can help to decrease soreness (making it the *only* proven thing you can do to prevent soreness other than taking your workout easier), lower your risk of injury, and even make your workout feel easier. If you do have time, postworkout is a great time to get in some stretching because your muscles are warm and pliable.

FAT BLAST MINUTE INTERVALS

Workout time: 15 to 19 minutes (20 to 26 minutes with warmup and cooldown)

Workout overview: After warming up with 3 to 5 minutes at an easy pace of the activity you'll be doing for your workout, pick it up to a moderately hard (but not gut-busting) pace—about a 7 or 8 on the 1 to 10 scale (see "Quick Guide to RPE" on page 107). Maintain the elevated pace for 1 minute, then slow it down for 1 minute to recover. If you're just starting out, do eight 1-minute pickups. As you get fitter, increase to 9, then 10 fast intervals. Cool down with a couple minutes of easy cardio.

And remember, while these workouts are designed to challenge you, they're also designed to be done at a level that you can handle. It's normal to be breathing hard, sweating, and feeling a little burn in your muscles. If you begin to feel dizzy, nauseated, or so out of breath that you can't talk at all, that's a sign to back off (and maybe even stop altogether) to give your body a chance to regroup.

ACTIVITY	TIME	EFFORT LEVEL
Warmup	0:00–5:00	4–5
Interval 1	5:00–6:00	7–8
Recovery	6:00–7:00	5–6
Interval 2	7:00–8:00	7–8
Recovery	8:00–9:00	5–6
Interval 3	9:00–10:00	7–8
Recovery	10:00–11:00	5–6
Interval 4	11:00–12:00	7–8
Recovery	12:00–13:00	5–6
Interval 5	13:00–14:00	7–8
Recovery	14:00–15:00	5–6
Interval 6	15:00–16:00	7–8
Recovery	16:00–17:00	5–6
Interval 7	17:00–18:00	7–8
Recovery	18:00–19:00	5–6
Interval 8	19:00–20:00	7–8
Recovery	20:00–21:00	5–6
Interval 9	21:00–22:00	7–8
Recovery	22:00–23:00	5–6
Interval 10	23:00–24:00	7–8
Cooldown	24:00–26:00	4–5

FAT BLAST 30-SECOND INTERVALS

Workout time: 14 to 27.5 minutes (19 to 34.5 minutes with warmup and cooldown)

Workout overview: After warming up with 3 to 5 minutes at an easy pace of the activity you'll be doing for your workout, alternate 30 seconds at an effort of 8 or 9 on a scale of 1 to 10 (see "Quick Guide to RPE" on page 107) with 4 minutes at a slow, comfortable pace. (If you need to, it's okay to stop altogether to catch your breath. Just don't sit down.) If you're just starting with the program, begin with just four fast 30-second intervals (14 minutes). Work up to seven total fast intervals

(27 minutes and 30 seconds). Finish with a few minutes of easy cardio until your heart rate gets back to normal.

ACTIVITY	TIME	EFFORT LEVEL
Warmup	0:00–5:00	4–5
Interval 1	5:00–5:30	8–9
Recovery	5:30–9:30	4–5
Interval 2	9:30–10:00	8–9
Recovery	10:00–14:00	4–5
Interval 3	14:00–14:30	8–9
Recovery	14:30–18:30	4–5
Interval 4	18:30–19:00	8–9
Recovery	19:00–23:00	4–5
Interval 5	23:00–23:30	8–9
Recovery	23:30–27:30	4–5
Interval 6	27:30–28:00	8–9
Recovery	28:00–32:00	4–5
Interval 7	32:00–32:30	8–9
Cooldown	32:30–34:30	4–5

AB BLAST SHORTCUT 8-SECOND INTERVALS

Workout time: 5 to 20 minutes (15 to 30 minutes with warmup and cooldown)

Workout overview: After at least 5 minutes of warming up, go as fast as you can for 8 seconds. (You'll need an especially thorough warmup for this workout because the sprints are short and all-out.) Slow your pace (or stop) for 12 seconds, then pick it up again, alternating 8 seconds fast with 12 seconds slow. When you first try this workout, start with about 15 intervals of fast/slow (5 minutes of high intensity). As you get fitter and stronger, add a few more intervals each time, working up to 60 interval cycles, or 20 minutes of intensity (30 minutes, including a 5-minute warmup and a 5-minute cooldown).

ACTIVITY	TIME	EFFORT LEVEL
Warmup	0:00–5:00	4–5
Interval 1	5:00–5:08	9–10
Recovery	5:08–5:20	4–5
Interval 2	5:20–5:28	9–10
Recovery	5:28–5:40	4–5
Interval 3	5:40–5:48	9–10
Recovery	5:48–6:00	4–5
Interval 4	6:00–6:08	9–10
Recovery	6:08–6:20	4–5
Interval 5	6:20–6:28	9–10
Recovery	6:28–6:40	4–5
Interval 6	6:40–6:48	9–10
Recovery	6:48–7:00	4–5
Interval 7	7:00–7:08	9–10
Recovery	7:08–7:20	4–5
Interval 8	7:20–7:28	9–10
Recovery	7:28–7:40	4–5
Interval 9	7:40–7:48	9–10
Recovery	7:48–8:00	4–5
Interval 10	8:00–8:08	9–10
Recovery	8:08–8:20	4–5
Interval 11	8:20–8:28	9–10
Recovery	8:28–8:40	4–5
Interval 12	8:40–8:48	9–10
Recovery	8:48–9:00	4–5
Interval 13	9:00–9:08	9–10
Recovery	9:08–9:20	4–5
Interval 14	9:20–9:28	9–10
Recovery	9:28–9:40	4–5
Interval 15	9:40–9:48	9–10
Recovery	9:48–10:00	4–5
Cooldown	10:00–15:00	4–5

FLAB FIGHTER 4-MINUTE INTERVALS

Workout time: 30 minutes (37 minutes with warmup and cooldown)

Workout overview: After warming up with 3 to 5 minutes at an easy pace of the activity you'll be doing for your workout, pick it up to a moderately hard (but not gut-busting) pace—about a 7 or 8 on the 1 to 10 scale. (See "Quick Guide to RPE" on page 107.) Maintain the elevated pace for 4 minutes, then slow it down for 2 minutes to recover. Aim to do five 4-minute pickups. If you have more time, bump it up for an extra challenge. Cool down with a couple minutes of easy cardio.

ACTIVITY	TIME	EFFORT LEVEL
Warmup	0:00–5:00	4–5
Interval 1	5:00–9:00	7–8
Recovery	9:00–11:00	4–5
Interval 2	11:00–15:00	7–8
Recovery	15:00–17:00	4–5
Interval 3	17:00–21:00	7–8
Recovery	21:00–23:00	4–5
Interval 4	23:00–27:00	7–8
Recovery	27:00–29:00	4–5
Interval 5	29:00–33:00	7–8
Recovery	33:00–35:00	4–5
Cooldown	35:00–37:00	4–5

20-MINUTE POWER BLAST

Workout time: 20 minutes (25 minutes with warmup and cooldown)

Workout overview: This routine is modeled after the University of Virginia study we talked about earlier, in which women shed five times as much belly fat from boosting their intensity and keeping it up. After warming up with 3 to 5 minutes at an easy pace of the activity you'll be doing for your workout, pick it up to a harder-than-usual pace, but one that you can maintain for 20 minutes. This is a good workout to test how much fitter you're getting if you do the same loop and try to go a little bit farther each time, or go out 10 minutes and try to make it back faster. One great way to motivate: Pick a local road race and do the workout there.

ACTIVITY	TIME	EFFORT LEVEL
Warmup	0:00–3:00	4–5
20-Minute Power	3:00–23:00	7–8
Cooldown	23:00–25:00	4–5

Your Choice Cardio

Feeling overwhelmed by all the cardio options or simply looking to try something new? Even something as seemingly simple as walking for exercise can be intimidating if you don't know where to start. Here's a little 411 on some of the most popular aerobic exercises you can do on this plan, including their benefits, ways to increase the intensity (it's not always all about speed!), and some insider tips.

Walking

Calories burned per hour: 225 (20 minutes per mile) to 544 (12 minutes per mile)

Why it's good: If you've ever read an issue of *Prevention* magazine, you probably know that we love walking. We're hardly alone. In fact, there are an astounding 108.7 million fitness walkers in the United States, according to the Sporting Goods Manufacturers Association, an industry group that keeps tabs on sports participation. It's also the exercise of choice among members of the National Weight Control Registry, a group made up of adults who have successfully lost an average of 66 pounds and kept it off for more than 5 years. Walking has been shown to decrease symptoms of depression, improve sleep, and increase insulin sensitivity as effectively as drugs (or even more so). And it's virtually injuryproof. Research shows that racewalkers on average suffer just one injury in more than 6 years of walking (or half that often for injuries severe enough to require taking a break from walking). Logging just 75 minutes a week may cut your risk of developing arthritis symptoms by 28 percent, while twice that could halve your risk, thanks to increased circulation that helps keep joints lubricated. Can you tell why we're fans?

How to do it: Okay, I know, you probably learned how to walk when you were around a year old. But walking for exercise, which typically means you'll be going faster and farther than you may be used to, does come with a bit of an instruction manual. I had been writing about fitness for years (and walking successfully for decades) when a meeting with Lee Scott, a walking coach in Toronto, delivered a true "aha" moment I've reached back to ever since when "teaching" exercisers how to walk. We were walking in Central Park in New York City (naturally when you meet with a walking coach, you do it on foot) and Lee had me walk "normally," then try bending my elbows to 90 degrees while I did it. Hello, power walker! While I can explain till I'm blue in the face why bending your elbows as you swing your arms creates a shorter lever that moves faster (blah blah blah), there is no replacement for simply trying it. Not only do you instantly "feel" like a walker—stronger and more powerful—but you also truly can walk faster! In fact, I soon found myself bending my elbows when I was late to get somewhere and rushing. Here are a few more tips for walking with good form.

- ○ **Mind your posture.** Looking up or down as you walk can throw off your alignment (it's okay to peek, just don't stare at the sidewalk or the sky). Keep your abs engaged so your back is supported, drop your shoulders away from your ears, and think about your ankle, knee, hip, and shoulder all stacking as you take a step.

- ○ **Practice running arms.** Overthinking the arm swing can make it start to feel unnatural—but it's not, I promise! Just think about running (or jog a couple steps). Notice how you automatically bend your arms? Now maintain that form for walking: Elbows stay bent at 90 degrees, swinging forward in opposition with your legs (when your right foot goes forward, your left arm will swing forward as well). Your hand should swing in an arc from your hip to the middle of your chest.

- ○ **Limit your strides.** It can be tempting to take bigger steps when you want to speed up, but doing so can actually slow you down and increase the stress on your legs. That's because big strides force your heel to act like a brake, stopping hard when you come down rather than smoothly rolling forward and spreading out the impact before you push off with your toes.

How to increase the intensity: Speed is, of course, the most obvious choice, and following the tips above can help you to increase your pace. Alternating running and walking is another great way to play with intensity whether or not you have a goal of becoming a full-time runner. But don't forget hills. Simply head uphill to increase the effort during your intervals, and walk back down during the recovery intervals. You can stick to the time guidelines in the workouts earlier in the chapter, or let the hill be your guide, walking up and then catching your breath on the way back down.

Running

Calories burned per hour: 544 (12 minutes per mile) to 850 (8 minutes per mile)

Why it's good: Running shares many of the same benefits as walking, with an added dose of higher impact because, unlike walking, where one foot is always on the ground, in running you actually push completely off the ground with each stride. A common misconception is that high impact is harmful. In fact, it's quite the opposite. While runners have an admittedly higher injury rate than walkers, that impact adds up to a relatively greater calorie burn per mile and stronger bones. When you strength train, your muscle fibers get damaged, then heal stronger than before. The same thing happens with bones. The pavement pounding of running adds up to greater bone density (at least in the lower body). Another busted misconception: Casual running does not wreck your knees or cause osteoarthritis, and it may even have a protective effect, concludes research on the topic. The one exception: Running through injury can exacerbate symptoms.

How to do it: Many of the same form guidelines listed for walking apply here. You still want your ankles, knees, hips, and shoulders to be in a stack, with your gaze looking out about 10 to 30 feet into the distance. The biggest difference from walking is in how you land on each step. Whereas walkers land heel first, runners should try to land on the middle of the foot, which allows the stress to be best dispersed.

If you aren't already a runner, beginning with walk-run intervals is a great way to start. Gradually increase the amount of time you spend running and decrease the time walking until you can run the full workout (if that's your goal).

How to increase the intensity: The same rules apply as with walking: Speed and hills are your best tools for tweaking intensity.

Swimming

Calories burned per hour: 544 to 748

Why it's good: Swimming might just be the ultimate anti-aging workout. In a 30-year study of more than 40,000 adults ages 20 to 90, swimmers were 50 percent less likely to die than sedentary peers or those who walked or ran. The University of South Carolina researchers suggest that swimming's prowess may have been a result of its very low injury risk combined with full-body strengthening thanks to the built-in resistance of water. Just being underwater provides 12 times more resistance than air every time you move. Taking a plunge is also a perfect indoor option in the winter, as well as a great way to beat the heat during the dog days of summer.

How to do it: As long as you know how to swim a simple front crawl or freestyle stroke, that's all you really need to get started. But if you're feeling out of practice, ask around about adult swimming programs at your local pool, YMCA, or community center. Even if they don't have anything on the roster, you might be able to find an instructor willing to give you some pointers. In fact, I've found that many lifeguards have a background in competitive swimming, and if the pool isn't busy, they're often more than willing to watch your form and make suggestions. And don't forget to wear goggles—a must for swimming in a straight line (there are usually lines on the bottom of the pool that you can follow to make sure you're going straight).

If you're swimming laps in a busy pool, some etiquette know-how can be helpful. It's okay to share a lane with someone else, but try to space it out, especially if you're swimming at a similar pace. Driving rules apply in the pool as well: Stick to the right-hand side of the lane unless you're passing, which you do on the left.

How to increase the intensity: As always, increasing your speed will increase the intensity, but paddling, stroking, or kicking faster isn't the only way to pick up the pace underwater. Stronger strokes, where you're really focusing on keeping your palm flat and pressing against as much water as possible, will also propel you faster and bump up the effort. For variety, you can experiment with some of the equipment on the pool deck that may be available for use. Flippers, for example, will create more resistance on your legs so they have to work harder. You may also find hand paddles that increase the surface area on your palm so your arms feel more resistance. And finally, holding a kickboard either with your arms or squeezing it between your legs allows the opposite part of the body to do all the work, creating an extra challenge.

Cardio Machines

Calories burned per hour: 476 to 612

Why they're good: Whether you have an elliptical machine in your basement or a gym with access to a full range of steppers and climbers, cardio machines insulate your workout from variables like weather, daylight, and traffic. Machines are generally very safe because they put you through a controlled range of motion, and they're low impact. They also make a darn good excuse for watching bad TV while you exercise. (Yes, this advice differs from what I told you in the strength chapter; while you don't want to zone out so much that you forget to keep your effort up, some folks find that distraction helps them to push themselves harder during cardio workouts.)

How to do it: While most machines come programmed with a variety of workouts, usually it just takes a couple presses of the "quick start" (or similar) button to put you in the driver's seat. The more information you program in (such as your weight and age), the more accurate the calorie burn estimate it gives you will be. But regardless, take it with a grain of salt as machines are notorious for being way off in their calculations.

The number one thing to remember as you're stepping, striding, or pedaling away on your machine of choice is to make sure that you're doing the work and not just taking a ride. While elliptical machines, for example, can give you a great workout, it's also easy to spend 30 minutes on one with little to show for it if you let the machine's momentum propel the pedals for you, allowing your legs to just float through the movements. Listen to your body to gauge how hard you're working, and adjust the machine's resistance as needed along with your own turnover, or foot speed, until you get a good effort going. And make sure to use your arms. If your machine has movable handles, use them. Otherwise, pump your arms at your sides just like you would when walking or running to increase your calorie burn.

How to increase the intensity: There are two variables you can control on most cardio machines: how fast you move your feet (or your arms), and how high you've set the resistance. If you go too fast with too little resistance, your legs will end up flying with little effort. Pump the resistance too high and you might feel yourself grind to a halt. A happy medium is best. To motivate yourself even as you're moving in place, use the numbers on the display—for example, setting goals of how much distance you can cover before each interval is over.

Bicycling

Calories burned per hour: 374 to 680

Why it's good: Biking offers similar benefits to walking and running, but it's a great alternative for folks with limitations (like painful joints) that make weight-bearing exercise uncomfortable. Outdoor cycling is also great for speed demons, because you can travel a lot faster and pass more scenery than you can on foot—no boredom here! Depending on where you live, it can also be a great way to get to work, making your workout that much more efficient (and saving gas and parking costs while you're at it).

How to do it: Start by setting the seat high enough that your "down" leg is not quite straight when the ball of your foot is on the pedal. This puts your body in the best ergonomic position on the bike, so needless aches and pains don't get in the way of your workout. (Bike shorts with padded bottoms, while a bit diaperlike, can help in this department too.)

Try to keep your pedaling rate to about 70 to 90 rotations per minute (rpm), adjusting the gears (for outdoor cycling) or the resistance (stationary bikes) to find a comfortable level. This helps to maximize the bloodflow to the legs, which in turn keeps the muscles energized so you can keep the effort up.

Don't forget a helmet if you're riding outdoors! Unlike walking or running, where you travel against the flow of traffic or on sidewalks, bicycles are usually prohibited from sidewalks and required to travel with the flow of traffic, or on the right-hand side of the road. Use the bike lane or shoulder if there is one, but avoid weaving in and out of the road, even if that means cars have to go around you. And remember: Traffic rules do apply to you, so stop at lights and stop signs, and give pedestrians the right of way. If your town has a local cycling or triathlon club, joining up for some practices can be a good opportunity to learn from more experienced riders. A bike repair shop should have information on nearby organizations or events.

How to increase the intensity: To boost intensity on a bike, you'll want to increase both your turnover (your pedal speed) and the resistance on the bike, which together is your "power" output. On a stationary bike, you might be able to see your power output as a number in watts. For outdoor cycling, a combination of these two things (a higher gear, which increases the resistance on the pedals, combined with slightly faster pedaling) is what will propel you forward faster. Indoors, increasing the resistance and pedaling faster will just give you a better workout.

Common Questions about Cardio Workouts

Q **I heard that low-intensity exercise burns more fat, but you're telling me the opposite. What gives?**

A Ah, the myth of the "fat-burning zone." There is a grain of truth behind that theory, which you still see emblazoned across cardio machine screens, but that doesn't mean you should slow down to slim down. When you exercise slowly, your body does actually burn proportionately more fat than carbohydrate, which is why there was a time when exercise scientists believed that was the best way to lose weight. However, when you're creeping along at a low intensity, you're not burning much of anything!

Instead of trying to burn more calories than fat during a 30-minute session, a better bet is to incorporate workouts that burn as many total calories—and as much fat—as possible, counting both during and after the workout. With that goal in mind, today's research shows that higher intensity is where it's at.

Q **I'm still having trouble figuring out what intensity I should be working out at for my Moderate Cardio workouts. Are there any other tricks to try to make sure I'm working hard enough—but not too hard?**

A Good question! I've always recommended a quick and easy estimate called the Talk Test, and as though on cue, some researchers at the University of Wisconsin–La Crosse just published a study for which they put this simple intensity gauge to the test. They found that difficulty in reciting the Pledge of Allegiance was just as good an indicator of exercisers' effort as was heavy-duty lab equipment like blood tests and masks that measured exactly what the exercisers breathed in and out. During your moderate intensity workouts, you should be able to say the pledge with a bit of effort or carry on a conversation with your workout buddy. If you can't, you're working too hard (save it for an Intensity day!). If you can sing the pledge, you need to kick it up a notch.

Can I do these workouts with my dog?

If your dog is anything like mine, he'll be so psyched to join you that he won't know how to contain himself. And that excitement can be contagious—it's hard to say no to those big brown eyes, after all. I'm hardly alone—several of the women who test-drove this program did it with canines in tow. Plenty of studies show that dog owners walk more, which can mean greater weight loss. Moderate Cardio workouts are a perfect opportunity to take almost any type of pup with you. But depending on what breed of dog you have and how old he is, he may or may not be good company for Intensity Cardio workouts. Personally, I try to jog or walk my 2-year-old Lab mix daily, and the little speed demon could leave me in the dust any day of the week; but I leave him home when I do intervals because I find it's easier to focus on pushing myself when I don't have a leash to worry about.

I was thinking of joining a women's soccer league. Does that count as Intensity or Moderate Cardio?

Because soccer involves a lot of stop-and-go sprints, it can absolutely count as an Intensity interval workout—as long as you're going after the ball and not standing on the sidelines, that is. In fact, researchers at the University of Copenhagen compared former couch potatoes who either started a steady-paced jogging routine or played soccer three times a week, and found some interesting results: The soccer set lost an average of nearly 6 pounds of fat over 12 weeks of training whereas joggers lost just 3 pounds of fat. The ball chasers also increased their rate of fat burning during a later jogging session, built stronger muscles and bones, and decreased their LDL ("bad") cholesterol. Perhaps it's not so surprising if you think about how similar the sprints up and down the field can be to more regimented interval workouts. But there's one other bonus with making your workout a game: The soccer players in the study rated their workouts as easier than the joggers did, possibly because they were so focused on the ball that they forgot how hard they were working!

Q I'm doing a lot of yard work this time of year. Does that count for my Moderate Cardio exercise?

A I'll give you a rousing "it depends!" First of all, anything you do that involves getting up and moving around instead of sitting on a couch or at a desk automatically doubles your calorie burn. But whether it counts as exercise depends on what you're doing. Pushing a lawn mower and raking leaves—as long as your heart is pumping faster than normal—count. Riding a lawn mower or sitting down pulling weeds, not so much. But it's still best to think of these activities as "extra credit" rather than the bread and butter of your routine. Also, if your goal is weight loss, you'll need to step it up from what your body is already used to. In other words, if you're trading TV for tomato growing, you may stand to benefit, whereas if the garden (or other household chores) has always been in your schedule, continuing with it only maintains the status quo. You have to do more than your body is accustomed to doing in order to lose.

Q I get a pain in my side sometimes when I run. Is there anything I can do?

A Ah, side stitches, stickers, whatever you want to call them, they're no fun! This stabbing side pain has perplexed runners, walkers, swimmers—and exercise researchers—for years. In fact, one study from a team of Australian researchers published in the journal *Medicine & Science in Sports & Exercise* found that this type of pain affects as many as 75 percent of exercisers at one time or another. There are a few theories on what causes them, from jostling organs to dehydration and poor posture, and even more suggested "treatments." You never know which will work for you, so try 'em all till you find something that helps (or until the stitch goes away on its own).

○ **Experiment with water.** Dehydration can leave you prone to muscle cramps, which may explain the pain in your side, but so can drinking too much too soon before exercise. Try having a big glass of water at least an hour before your workout, and no more than small sips right before.

○ **Even your breathing.** An old trick passed down through the ranks of side stitch sufferers is to time your breathing with your steps—exhaling hard when the foot opposite the stitch strikes and in when the other foot lands. Breathing every step might be too fast, depending on your pace, so find a tempo that feels comfortable (I tend to get an every-other rhythm going). There may or may not be any magic to that exact sequence, but the simple act of focusing on and steadying your breathing seems to help some people.

○ **Press into the pain.** A jab with your fingers into the spot that hurts can sometimes help, combined with a sharp exhale. Bending over to touch your toes can have a similar effect (my personal go-to fix).

○ **Stand up straight!** In a recent study, the same team of Australian researchers demonstrated that exercisers with side cramps were more likely to be running with hunched-over posture than were their cramp-free counterparts. To straighten up your running (or walking) form, imagine that there is a straight line striking through your body from your ankles to your hips, shoulders, and ears. Now take that line and tip it forward slightly from the ankles (not the waist). Relax your hands, drop your shoulders, and gaze out at the horizon, rather than at the ground in front of your feet. Ahhh.

Q I've been walking regularly for years and I'm raring to go. Can I do more Intensity Cardio workouts than the plan recommends?

A In short, yes. This plan was designed to be doable for readers of all different levels, so if you're already pretty aerobically fit, you might be ready to step it up faster to two or three Intensity workouts a week sooner than the plan suggests (if you choose). You can always do as much Moderate Cardio as you like. The important thing is that you don't get so carried away with cardio that you find yourself lapsing on the strength workouts. If you're a regular cardiophile, you may find you have to decrease the time you spend on those workouts to make time for resistance training, and that's okay. Above all, listen to your body. If you're feeling excessively tired or sore, back it off before you find yourself with an injury that requires you to stop altogether.

Keeping a Record

Just like with the strength workouts in Chapters 3 and 4, keeping track of what days you did cardio; which Intensity workouts you did; how you felt; and other details like how far you went, how many intervals you completed, and how fast you walked, biked, swam, or ran can help you to see your progress as you get fitter and stronger. Unlike your strength log, however, there's no need to have a different log for every day you do cardio. Instead, I recommend using the following log to track all of your workouts—cardio and strength—in one place over the course of the week. (Because you have a separate, more detailed log for each strength workout, you only need to note here that you did a strength workout.)

Being able to see your whole week of exercise at a glance will also help you to spot trends in order to work out a routine that works best for you. For example, if doing strength workouts the day before cardio intervals leaves you sore, maybe you'll decide to rearrange the week so there's a day off or a Moderate Cardio day in between. There's a sample log on the next page, and you'll also find a blank form to photocopy on page 308 in the Tone Every Inch Logs.

Weekly Exercise Overview

Week of program: 3   **Date:** 3/18/12

DAY	WORKOUTS	TIME OF DAY	DURATION	OBSERVATIONS/ CHALLENGES	DAILY TOTAL EXERCISE TIME
Mon.	Fat Blast Minute Intervals (8)	5:30 p.m.	23 min.	Really pushed myself. Felt great after!	23 min.
Tues.	Strength workout	noon	30 min.	A little sore from yesterday's interval workout. But getting stronger!	30 min.
Wed.	Off				
Thurs.	Strength workout	noon	30 min.		30 min.
Fri.	Off				
Sat.	Fat Blast 30-Second Intervals (4 with 4 min. break)	8 a.m.	25 min.	Made it around the neighborhood loop in 28 minutes today.	25 min.
Sun.	Walk	4 p.m.	60 min.	Long walk with Nancy and had a good catch-up session.	60 min.

Donna Holzbaur

Age 46

Lost: 11 percent body fat

Gained: Confidence at the gym

Favorite move: Cheerleader Press

Donna Holzbaur could no longer blame lack of time for keeping her from exercising. Thanks to a new job with an hour-long lunch break and convenient access to an employee fitness center, Donna was ready to start the new year by turning over a new leaf. The question now was where to start. "I would feel uncomfortable going to the gym because I didn't know what to do," says the novice exerciser, who had never dared to go near weights before. Donna had joined various gyms in the past but never found anything she'd stick with for more than a short time. She had just signed up for the fitness center at work when she noticed an advertisement for the Tone Every Inch study, and it seemed like just the dose of structure she needed. Her modest goal for the program: to finally stick with a fitness program long enough to see results.

Part of the reason exercise had never stuck was that Donna had never seen results from working out before. She'd also never tried any sort of strength training—bands, dumbbells, or otherwise. This time, tangible benefits gave her a boost right off the bat. "With the band workout, I felt stronger and could feel that it was working," Donna says. "That was motivating." Sure enough, in just the first 3 weeks of the program she increased her leg strength by 15 percent, and by the end of 8 weeks she'd increased her upper-body strength by 12.5 percent as well. "Before the study, I was never an exercise person," she admits. But by the end of Week 3, the workouts had become something she really *wanted* to do.

As a lunchtime exerciser, one barrier Donna had to find a way to navigate was making sure a growling stomach didn't talk her out of her workout. "Sometimes I would get so hungry that I would choose to eat, and then blow off exercising," she says. Learning to eat something small, like Chobani Greek yogurt, preworkout was an easy solution.

Meanwhile, the loss of 5 pounds of fat along with an increase in lean muscle mass reduced Donna's body fat percentage by 11 percent. But perhaps best of all, by braving the gym regularly armed with a game plan of strength and cardio, she gained confidence in using the equipment and the space. And while she'd never found exercise to be fun before, experimenting with different types of workouts on cardio days led her to Zumba, which, surprise, was genuinely a blast. Feeling the effects of her strength gains was another incentive to stick with exercise. "I did some pushups yesterday, and I was surprised that I felt really strong doing them," she says. "It shocked me!" By the end of 8 weeks, the former nonexerciser had left the building.

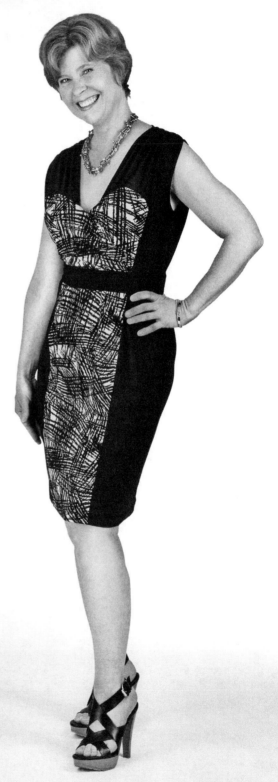

The Lighten-Up 7-Day Kickstart Menu

Slow and steady wins the race. Patience is a virtue. You've heard these adages a million times; nevertheless, there's no better motivation than seeing pounds disappear right away. And the latest research suggests that the motivational boost of losing weight quickly—at least at the start of a new program—actually translates to more weight lost and doesn't leave you more susceptible to the dreaded regain. When scientists at the University of Florida in Gainesville tracked 262 obese middle-aged women who lost weight through a diet and exercise program, they found that the fastest initial losers were five times more likely to achieve a loss of at least 10 percent of their starting body weight (a benchmark commonly used by researchers because it's been shown to provide sizable health benefits). And they weren't any more likely than their more turtlelike counterparts to gain the weight back.

With that in mind, we created this special Lighten-Up 7-Day Kickstart eating plan for the Tone Every Inch program to make sure you see results right away—even as your workouts are still getting up to speed (the first week of the exercise plan is focused on learning the new exercises). Although following this diet for the duration of the program wouldn't give you the energy and nutrition you'll need as your workouts advance through the plan, following it for 1 week is just enough to get you off the ground and running. For tester Merry Buckley, who dropped nearly 4 pounds in the first week alone thanks to the Kickstart, a successful start launched her into a total of 11 pounds down and counting by the end of the program. And when she saw the number on the scale, she could hardly believe it. "I've never been in the habit of weighing myself before and have never been much of a mindful eater," she says, adding that she was surprised by the low number. But it was just the incentive she needed to head into the next 7 weeks of the program, confident that she'd see results.

The Kickstart Principles

The 7 days' worth of menus in this chapter are designed to provide all the balanced nutrition you need to get started on this program, reduce your calorie intake while still helping you to feel full and energized, and decrease bloating so you feel slimmer and less sluggish right away. Here's how it works:

- ○ Each day you'll eat three meals plus a snack, totaling 1,200 calories.
- ○ You'll have a maximum of 1,500 milligrams sodium and minimum of 2,300 milligrams potassium per day to regulate water balance and beat bloating.
- ○ You'll limit your saturated fat intake to no more than 10 percent of your calories, or no more than 12 grams per day, because saturated fat tends to be stored more readily as body fat.
- ○ Each meal will contain at least 8 grams of fiber to help you feel full.
- ○ You'll get 20 grams of protein from each meal and 15 grams from each snack to fuel muscle strengthening.
- ○ You'll drink 8 cups (64 ounces) of water each day to help flush out toxins, carry nutrients to your cells, and prevent dehydration-triggered lethargy.
- ○ Each breakfast offers a "Breakaway Breakfast" option with about 15 grams of carbohydrate to allow you to munch something first thing if you plan to do an a.m. workout.

Potassium and Sodium: The Keys to Banishing Bloat

Eating fewer calories isn't the only way to drop extra pounds. Balancing the amounts of sodium and potassium you eat—two dietary minerals that regulate fluid retention in your body—will also go a long way to beating puffiness and bloating so you look and feel lighter fast.

Potassium is the principal positive-charge ion in the fluid inside of your cells, while sodium is the principal positive-charge ion in the fluid outside of your cells. By increasing your potassium intake and decreasing your sodium intake, the concentration differences between potassium and sodium across your cell membranes push sodium out of the

Did You Know? Bloat-Busting Foods

In addition to busting extra water weight, studies show that getting enough potassium decreases your risk for osteoporosis, hypertension, and stroke. The following foods can help you up your intake.

FOOD	SERVING	AMOUNT OF POTASSIUM (MG)
Baked potato	1 medium	1,081
Kale	2 cups raw	599
Banana	1 medium	594
Yogurt	8 ounces	579
Cantaloupe	1 cup	494
Dried apricots	7 halves	490
Lima beans	½ cup	485
Tomato sauce	½ cup	453
Winter squash	½ cup	448
Dried plums	7 whole	406
Fat-free milk	1 cup	382
Spinach	2 cups raw	335
Beets	¾ cup	330
Asparagus	8 medium spears	259
Orange	1 medium	237

cells and potassium into the cells, which cues excess water from the cells in your body to get the heck out of Dodge. More accurately, the extra water flees to the bloodstream, gets filtered out by your kidneys, and leaves the body. How much of a difference this will make varies from person to person, but it could account for a loss of up to 5 or 6 pounds.

All about Water

How's this for a contradiction: To make sure you're not lugging around 5 extra pounds of water weight, you may actually need to drink more water. That's right. Your body is great at clinging to whatever resources it thinks are scarce, including good old H_2O. If you stop drinking enough, your body starts hoarding. We recommend aiming for about 64 ounces of water a day, or 8 cups, to keep everything "flowing," so to speak, but you might want more if you sweat a lot during your workouts. An easy way to do it: Have 2 cups (or one tall glass) with every meal plus your snack. Bonus: It'll also help you feel full faster, buffering the gap between when your stomach and your brain realize you've had enough to eat.

The Power of Protein

Protein tends to get a bad rap, thanks to its association with grease-dripping cheeseburgers and the like, perhaps the reason that statistics from the US Department of Agriculture show that as many as one-third of women don't get enough. Especially when you're trying to sculpt muscle (and minimize age-related muscle shrinking), protein is essential for repairing and rebuilding the muscle tissue you break down by working out, shaping it into stronger, firmer, more metabolically active muscles than before.

Protein is also one of the most important foods in your weight loss arsenal for a couple of reasons. First of all, let's set something straight: Protein packs the exact same number of calories per gram as carbohydrate—4. (Fat, on the other hand, contains a hefty 9 calories per gram—the reason such a teeny sliver of cheesecake can pack such a caloric wallop.) But it's more complicated than that. Protein-laden foods take more energy to break down and digest than do carbs,

> **⊃ Helpful Hints:** Deli Meats
>
> Along with being an easy and versatile sandwich stuffer and salad topper, deli meats (including turkey, chicken, ham, and even beef) can be an excellent source of lean protein. Their one dark side: sky-high sodium levels. Even seemingly safe sliced turkey can pack nearly 600 milligrams of sodium per serving. Luckily, brands vary widely, and lower-sodium varieties are increasingly available. To help you stay within the 1,500-milligram limit this week (as well as the 2,300-milligram guideline for the rest of the plan), look for a variety with no more than 480 milligrams per 2-ounce serving.

meaning you burn more calories just converting them into fuel your body can use. All that extra work in digestion also means the protein sticks around in your stomach, helping you to feel full longer.

Of course, a juicy steak is going to weigh in with a lot more calories than a carrot stick, but all sources of protein are not created equal. And remember, protein is just one "macronutrient" in nutrition-speak (the others are carbs and fat), and most foods are made up of some combination of the three. The protein isn't to blame for that steak

MEATLESS MUSCLE BUILDING

You may have heard the old vegetarian wisdom that meat-free proteins aren't complete unless you pair them with certain complementary foods (like rice and beans, or peanut butter and bread). Not so! I'm not knocking rice and beans—it's a great combo. But more recent research—enough of it to convince the American Dietetic Association to change its position on the subject—shows that as long as you eat a variety of plant-based foods over the course of the day, you can still get all the amino acids (or so-called building blocks of protein) that you need. So even if you have your beans for breakfast and your rice for dinner, the net effect will be the same as if you ate them together. Still, there are a few tips to keep in mind to make sure your meat-free lifestyle is as nutritious as it ought to be.

Don't be tricked by the health halo. While many vegetarian choices are lighter and leaner than their meaty counterparts, don't forget to keep an eye on fat and calories. For example, edamame beans, for all their green goodness, pack almost 200 calories per cup (not to mention all that salt that might be sprinkled on the outside).

Don't overdo meat substitutes. The vegetarian freezer section is stocked with a McDonald's menu's worth of imitation hamburgers, sausages, and chicken nuggets. A good veggie burger can go a long way to helping you BBQ with the best of them, and imitation meat products have being so calorically dense; the fat content is. So the key to upping the protein in your diet while downsizing your waistline is choosing lean protein sources that don't come with supersize servings of fat on the side. Fish, skinless poultry, and even lean beef and pork can be great options.

But meats are not the only way. In fact, we had several vegetarians (and vegetarians' wives who eat mostly meatless meals) on our test panel, and even one vegan. Beans, nuts, and dairy, and even some

even made it into a few of the recipes and meals in this book. But try not to rely on these as the foundation of your meals, as they can pack a surprising amount of sodium. Look for beans, quinoa, legumes, and nuts to supply most of the meatless protein on your plate.

Do go easy on the cheese. Like most milk products, cheese can be a good source of protein. But it's an even better source of saturated fat, something this plan aims to cut down on.

Do keep an eye out for vitamins and minerals you might be missing. In addition to protein, meat supplies some vital nutrients. Be sure to load up on vegetarian sources of these vitamins and minerals.

- **Vitamin B$_{12}$:** Find it in milk products, eggs, fortified cereals, meat substitutes, and soy drinks.

- **Iron:** Find it in dark leafy greens, whole wheat breads, kidney beans, lentils, and dried fruits like apricots, prunes, and raisins.

- **Calcium:** If you don't drink milk, find calcium in fortified cereals, tofu, dark leafy vegetables, and calcium-fortified milk substitutes such as soy, almond, rice, or hemp milk. Look for fortified foods with added vitamin D as well to help your body absorb the calcium.

- **Zinc:** Find it in white beans, kidney beans, garbanzo beans, pumpkin seeds, zinc-fortified breakfast cereals, and wheat germ.

grains, like quinoa, can provide a surprising amount of protein. It does take a bit more planning to get sufficient protein without meat (see "Meatless Muscle Building" on page 136 for tips), but you'll see plenty of options in the meals that start on page 146 for ways to get creative beyond grilled chicken.

Fill-You-Up Fiber

Similar to protein, fiber also puts the brakes on digestion, helping you to feel full longer. It steadies blood sugar, leveling out the spike/fall pattern that can cause energy crashes (leaving your brain foggy and you reaching for midafternoon cookies in a desperate effort to raise your blood sugar back up to normal levels). The result: more energy all day long, fewer binges, and feeling satisfied even while eating less. Sound good? Unfortunately, most Americans get an average of just

FIBERFUL FOODS

Beans, whole grains, fruits, and vegetables all provide fiber. Here's a list of some of the most common and best sources of fiber.

FOOD	SERVING	AMOUNT OF FIBER (G)
High-fiber cereal	½ cup	6–14
Lentils	¼ cup cooked	12
Beans (such as black beans, kidney beans, or chickpeas)	½ cup cooked or canned	6–8
Bran flakes cereal	¾ cup	5–6
Pear	1 medium	5
Apple	1 medium	4
Blueberries	1 cup	4
Oatmeal	1 cup prepared, or ½ cup dry	4
Whole wheat pasta	1 cup cooked	4
Broccoli	½ cup cooked	3

15 grams of fiber per day. For this plan, you'll aim for the USDA's recommendation of 25 grams. Each meal on the plan provides at least 8 grams, while each snack contributes at least 2, adding up to an easy 25 grams or more per day.

There are two different types of fiber you'll find in the food you eat—soluble and insoluble—and each type has its own list of benefits.

SOLUBLE FIBER

What it does: Traps carbohydrates in your digestive system and tempers absorption, slowing the release of sugar into your bloodstream. Soluble fiber also binds to cholesterol in the digestive tract before it can be absorbed, helping to lower cholesterol levels.

Best sources: Oats, fruits, and beans

INSOLUBLE FIBER

What it does: Hampers the absorption of dietary fat, which can help to shave off a few calories from your meal.

Best sources: Wheat bran, whole wheat, and veggies

Working On Your Schedule

If you work out first thing in the morning, you might be tempted to do so before breakfast. But eating something first is key to ensuring you have enough energy to get the most out of your workout and feel good doing it. You may have worked out on an empty stomach before and thought it was fine, but trust me and try it—you'll feel 10 times better with some fuel in the tank!

Of course, wolfing down an entire omelet right before your workout won't necessarily leave you feeling great either. The ideal recipe for an energized a.m. workout is about 15 grams of carbohydrate for a quick pick-me-up (depending on grams of protein or fat in your meal, this will be at least 100 calories, maybe more). You'll have to experiment to find out what works for you—a cup of yogurt works great for some folks, while pre-exercise dairy spells stomach cramps for others.

To get you started, the Breakaway Breakfast Option included in most of the breakfast menus and recipes both for the Kickstart and the general plan in Chapter 8 is a part of the meal that you can easily break off and eat right away before doing your workout. These options are designed to fuel your workout while being easy to eat and digest on the go. Once you're done with your workout, you'll go ahead and finish up the rest of the meal. (If you have a stomach of steel—lucky you—there's nothing wrong with eating the full breakfast pre-workout.)

The Lighten-Up 7-Day Kickstart Meal Plan

For this 7-Day Kickstart, each recipe or meal below is designed to serve one. While many of the recipes for the weeks that follow can easily be shared as a nutritious meal with your spouse or family, this part of the plan is dedicated to you, and the meals are formulated specifically to meet your needs and goals as a woman on this program. You'll get the maximum benefit if you follow the 7 days of meals given as closely as possible.

Here's the breakdown of the nutritional guidelines we followed for the Kickstart Phase, which lasts for 1 full week:

Per Day

- ○ 1,200 calories
- ○ 75 grams of protein minimum
- ○ 25 grams of fiber minimum
- ○ 1,500 milligrams of sodium maximum
- ○ 2,300 milligrams of potassium minimum
- ○ 8 cups (64 ounces) water
- ○ 12 grams of saturated fat maximum

Meal-by-Meal Breakdown

○ Breakfast: 300 calories with at least 8 grams of fiber and 20 grams of protein

○ Lunch: 300 calories with at least 8 grams of fiber and 20 grams of protein

○ Snack: 200 calories with at least 2 grams of fiber and 15 grams of protein

○ Dinner: 400 calories with at least 8 grams of fiber and 20 grams of protein

Lighten-Up 7-Day Kickstart Shopping List

The amounts listed on the following pages include exactly what you will use throughout the Kickstart. Use this as a checklist to make sure you have what you need. In some cases, you may have to buy a bit more of an ingredient than you need, but you may be able to use it later on in the meal plan.

If you need a small amount of an ingredient, consider buying from a bulk section of a store, where you can purchase exact amounts, or use the store salad bar for small amounts of produce.

Produce

Cantaloupe, 1 cup cubes

Spinach, one 10-ounce bag

Hass avocado, 1 small

Bananas, 2 medium

Asparagus, 10 medium spears or 1 small bag frozen

Lemon juice, 1 lemon or 1 small container lemon juice
(1 tablespoon)

Oranges, 1 medium and 1 large

Green bell pepper, 1 small (¼ cup chopped, about ½ pepper)

Red bell pepper, 1 small (¼ cup chopped, about ½ pepper)

Onion, 1 small, chopped (6 tablespoons, about ½ small onion)

Minced garlic, 6 teaspoons minced

Honeydew melon, ¾ cup chopped

Baby carrots, 1 cup

Kale, about 8 ounces, chopped (3 cups)

Raspberries, fresh, 1 pint (or 2¼ cups unsweetened frozen)

Kiwifruit, 6 small

Edamame, fresh or frozen shelled, ¾ cup

Broccoli florets, fresh, 1 cup (or frozen, about 4 ounces)

Cauliflower florets, fresh, ¾ cup (or frozen, about 4 ounces)

Carrots, fresh, ½ cup (or frozen, sliced, about 3 ounces)

Tofu, firm, 6 ounces

Tomato, 2 medium

Pear, 1 large

Nectarine or peach, 1 medium (or 1 cup unsweetened
frozen peach slices)

Mixed baby greens, one 8-ounce bag

Potato, russet or Yukon gold, 1 large

Romaine lettuce, 2 cups

Orange juice, 2 tablespoons

Grapes, ½ cup

Parsley, fresh, 1 tablespoon

Chives, chopped, 2 teaspoons

Dairy

Greek yogurt, 0%, plain, five 8-ounce containers

Fat-free milk, ½ gallon

Reduced-fat cream cheese, 1 tablespoon

Cottage cheese, 1% or fat-free, no-salt-added, 8 ounces (1 cup)

Mozzarella cheese, reduced-sodium, 1 ounce

Ricotta cheese, fat-free, 8 ounces

Cheddar cheese, 2% reduced-fat, shredded, 1 ounce (¼ cup)

Yogurt, fat-free, plain, 8 ounces (1 cup)

Eggs

Egg whites, 8 large (or egg substitute, 1 cup)

Frozen Foods

Spinach, chopped, ¾ cup (4 ounces)

Healthy Choice Complete Meals Beef Bourbon Dijon or Beef Tips Portobello

Corn, frozen, 1 cup (or 5 ounces)

Morningstar Farms Chik Patties, 1 patty

Bread/Cereal

Cereal with at least 6 grams of fiber per 100 calories (such as Kashi Good Friends or Barbara's Bakery Original), 1 cup

Whole wheat bread with 80 calories and 3 grams of fiber per slice (such as Martin's Whole Wheat Potato Bread or Weight Watchers 100 percent Whole Wheat Bread), 1 slice

Cereal with added protein (such as Kellogg's Special K Protein Plus or Kashi GoLean), 1½ cups

Whole wheat pita (8-inch), 1

Dry Goods

Cooking spray

Walnuts, chopped, 5 teaspoons

Balsamic vinegar, 5 tablespoons

Olive oil, 2 tablespoons + ½ teaspoon

Quinoa, ¼ cup dry

Rice vinegar or white vinegar, 4 tablespoons

Raisins, 4 tablespoons

Pasta, whole wheat, penne, ½ ounce dry

Pasta, whole wheat spaghetti, 1½ ounces dry

Whole wheat flatbread-style crackers with about 45 calories each (such as Wasa), 6

Apricot halves, dried, 6

Figs, dried, 1

Dates, 5

Chunk light tuna, no-salt-added water pack, one 6-ounce can

Wild or brown rice, 6 tablespoons dry

Stewed tomatoes, canned, no-salt-added, 8 ounces (1 cup)

Peanuts, 2 tablespoons

Sesame oil, 1½ teaspoons

Canola oil, 1 teaspoon

Spaghetti sauce with no more than 400 milligrams of sodium per ½ cup serving (such as Muir Glen), ½ cup

Chickpeas, no-salt-added canned, 2 ounces (¼ cup)

Pecans, 1 teaspoon

Vegetarian chili (such as Health Valley Organic No Salt Added Tame Tomato Chili), one 15.5-ounce can (1¾ cups)

Meat/Seafood

Turkey breast, deli sliced, with no more than 360 milligrams of sodium per 2-ounce serving (such as Applegate Farms or Boar's Head), 5 ounces

Roast beef, deli sliced, with no more than 320 milligrams of sodium per 2-ounce serving (such as Applegate Farms), 2 ounces

Ham, deli sliced, with no more than 480 milligrams of sodium per 2-ounce serving (such as Applegate Farms), 2 ounces

Salmon, 3 ounces raw (2 ounces cooked)

Chicken breast, boneless, skinless, 4 ounces raw (2 ounces cooked)

Ground beef, 90 percent lean, 3 ounces raw (2 ounces cooked)

Turkey breast tenderloin, 4 ounces raw (3 ounces cooked)

Spices and Seasonings

Vanilla extract, 1 teaspoon

Capers, 1 teaspoon

Dill, dried, ⅛ teaspoon

Sesame seeds, 2 tablespoons

Light soy sauce, 1 teaspoon

Dijon mustard, ½ teaspoon

Rosemary, dried, ½ teaspoon

Basil, dried, ½ teaspoon

Kickstart | Day 1

Breakfast

Crunchy Greek Yogurt and Cantaloupe

Have ¾ cup 0% plain Greek yogurt mixed with ¾ cup cereal (pick one with at least 6 grams of fiber per 100 calories, such as Kashi Good Friends or Barbara's Bakery Original). Serve with 1 cup cubed cantaloupe topped with 2 teaspoons chopped walnuts.

Breakaway Breakfast Option:

Eat the cantaloupe topped with chopped walnuts.

Per serving: 300 calories, 20 g protein, 53 g carbohydrates, 5 g total fat, 0.5 g saturated fat, 10 g fiber, 180 mg sodium, 646 mg potassium

Lunch

Avocado Spinach Salad

Top 4 cups baby spinach with one-eighth avocado, sliced, and 2 ounces thinly sliced low-sodium turkey breast (no more than 360 milligrams of sodium per 2-ounce serving). Drizzle with a splash of balsamic vinegar and ½ teaspoon olive oil. Serve with ¾ cup cooked quinoa tossed with 2 teaspoons rice vinegar and 1 teaspoon raisins.

Speed-it-up tip: Leftover cooked quinoa can be frozen and reheated when needed. Just sprinkle with water and microwave.

Per serving: 320 calories, 22 g protein, 41 g carbohydrates, 8 g total fat, 1 g saturated fat, 8 g fiber, 520 mg sodium, 1,038 mg potassium

Snack

Banana Smoothie

Blend 1⅔ cups fat-free milk with ½ cup sliced banana and ½ teaspoon vanilla extract.

Per serving: 210 calories, 15 g protein, 38 g carbohydrates, 1 g total fat, 0 g saturated fat, 2 g fiber, 170 mg sodium, 906 mg potassium

Dinner

Penne with Salmon and Capers

Toss ½ cup cooked whole wheat penne pasta with 2 ounces broiled salmon, flaked; 1½ teaspoons olive oil; 1 tablespoon chopped fresh parsley; and 1 teaspoon capers. Serve with 10 medium spears asparagus, steamed, and drizzle with a splash of lemon juice. Serve with 1 medium orange.

Per serving: 400 calories, 35 g protein, 43 g carbohydrates, 13 g total fat, 0 g saturated fat, 10 g fiber, 190 mg sodium, 1,061 mg potassium

Kickstart | Day 2

Breakfast

Primavera Scrambled Eggs

Coat a skillet with cooking spray and heat over medium heat. Add ¼ cup each chopped green bell pepper, red bell pepper, and onion. Cook until softened, about 3 minutes. Add ¾ cup or 6 large egg whites and 1 teaspoon fresh minced garlic. Cook, stirring, until the eggs are set. Serve with 3 multigrain flatbread-style crackers (for example, Wasa brand or similar with about 45 calories each), each spread with 1 teaspoon reduced-fat cream cheese and topped with 2 dried apricot halves.

Breakaway Breakfast Option:

Have 2 of the crackers spread with cream cheese
and topped with dried apricot halves.

Per serving: 335 calories, 18 g protein, 53 g carbohydrates, 3 g total fat, 1 g saturated fat, 10 g fiber, 596 mg sodium, 768 mg potassium

Lunch

Tuna and Honeydew Wrap

Toss 3 ounces no-salt-added chunk light tuna packed in water with 2 tablespoons 0% Greek yogurt, ⅛ teaspoon dried dill, and ¼ cup chopped honeydew. Roll up in a whole wheat wrap (with at least 6 grams of fiber and about 120 calories). Serve with a side of ½ cup honeydew cubes and 1 cup baby carrots.

Per serving: 310 calories, 29 g protein, 44 g carbohydrates, 5 g total fat, 1 g saturated fat, 10 g fiber, 590 mg sodium, 198 mg potassium

Snack

Fig and Nut Yogurt

Stir 1 fig, chopped, and 2 teaspoons chopped walnuts into ⅔ cup 0% Greek yogurt.

Per serving: 210 calories, 16 g protein, 14 g carbohydrates, 11 g total fat, 1 g saturated fat, 2 g fiber, 55 mg sodium, 133 mg potassium

Dinner

Chicken and Savory Kale

Coat a saucepan with cooking spray and heat over medium-low heat. Cook 2 tablespoons chopped onion for 2 minutes. Add 3 cups chopped kale, 1 teaspoon minced fresh garlic, and ½ teaspoon olive oil; reduce heat to low, cover, and continue cooking for 10 minutes, stirring occasionally. Serve with 3 ounces roasted chicken breast and ½ cup cooked wild rice tossed with ¼ cup raspberries (fresh or unsweetened frozen and thawed).

Per serving: 400 calories, 36 g protein, 44 g carbohydrates, 11 g total fat, 2.5 g saturated fat, 8 g fiber, 150 mg sodium, 1,277 mg potassium

Breakfast

Cereal and Fruit

In a bowl, top ¼ cup high-fiber cereal (pick one with at least 6 grams of fiber per 100 calories, such as Kashi Good Friends or Barbara's Bakery Original) with ½ cup fat-free milk. Have 1 cup 0% Greek yogurt and 2 sliced kiwifruits.

Breakaway Breakfast Option:

Eat the cereal and milk.

Per serving: 310 calories, 26 g protein, 49 g carbohydrates, 2 g total fat, 0 g saturated fat, 8 g fiber, 180 mg sodium, 728 mg potassium

Lunch

Garlic Spinach, Edamame, and Tomato

In a bowl, combine 1 cup no-salt-added canned stewed tomatoes, ¾ cup chopped frozen spinach, and 2 teaspoons each minced garlic and olive oil. Microwave on high power for 1 minute. Stir and heat for 30 seconds. Add ¾ cup fresh or frozen shelled edamame and heat until warmed through, about 1½ minutes.

Per serving: 310 calories, 20 g protein, 29 g carbohydrates, 16 g total fat, 2 g saturated fat, 13 g fiber, 190 mg sodium, 923 mg potassium

Snack

Peanuts, Raisins, and Cottage Cheese

Have 2 tablespoons peanuts and 2 teaspoons raisins. On the side, have ½ cup no-salt-added fat-free or 1% cottage cheese. You can stir the peanuts and raisins right into the cottage cheese, if desired.

Per serving: 210 calories, 20 g protein, 12 g carbohydrates, 10 g total fat, 2 g saturated fat, 2 g fiber, 15 mg sodium, 269 mg potassium

Dinner

Tofu and Veggie Stir-Fry

Heat 1½ teaspoons sesame oil in a nonstick skillet over medium heat. Add 1 cup frozen broccoli florets, ¾ cup frozen cauliflower florets, and ½ cup carrots, and cook for 5 minutes, stirring often. Add 6 ounces firm tofu, drained* and cubed; 2 tablespoons sesame seeds; 2 teaspoons minced garlic; and 1 teaspoon light soy sauce. Heat for 5 minutes, or until the tofu is cooked on all sides and the vegetables are warmed through. Serve over ½ cup cooked brown rice.

Per serving: 420 calories, 25 g protein, 44 g carbohydrates, 17 g total fat, 2.5 g saturated fat, 10 g fiber, 300 mg sodium, 790 mg potassium

*See page 239 for a tip on how to drain tofu.

Kickstart | Day 4

Breakfast

Grab-and-Go Cheese and Crackers

Have 2 multigrain flatbread-style crackers (Wasa brand or similar, about 45 calories each), each topped with ½ ounce reduced-sodium mozzarella cheese. Serve with 1 cup fat-free milk and 1 large orange.

Breakaway Breakfast Option:

Eat the orange.

Per serving: 314 calories, 21 g protein, 48 g carbohydrates, 5 g total fat, 3.5 g saturated fat, 7 g fiber, 267 mg sodium, 646 mg potassium

Lunch

Turkey Sandwich

Make a sandwich with 1 slice whole wheat bread (with at least 3 grams of fiber) and 3 ounces sliced low-sodium turkey breast (no more than 360 milligrams of sodium per 2-ounce serving) and 2 thick slices tomato. Have with 1 large pear.

Per serving: 272 calories, 23 g protein, 46 g carbohydrates, 1 g total fat, 0 g saturated fat, 9 g fiber, 714 mg sodium, 343 mg potassium

Snack

Fruit and Nut Ricotta Cheese

Have ⅔ cup fat-free ricotta cheese mixed with 1 nectarine, sliced, or 1 cup unsweetened frozen and thawed peach slices and 1 teaspoon chopped walnuts.

Per serving: 210 calories, 15 g protein, 29 g carbohydrates, 2 g total fat, 0 g saturated fat, 2 g fiber, 170 mg sodium, 467 mg potassium

Dinner

Spaghetti with Meat Sauce and Mixed Green Salad

Heat a saucepan over medium-low heat with 1 teaspoon canola oil. Cook 2 ounces of 90% lean ground beef (leaner beef is fine, too) until cooked through, 5 to 7 minutes. Toss together with ⅔ cup cooked whole wheat spaghetti and ½ cup spaghetti sauce (look for one with no more than 400 milligrams of sodium per ½-cup serving). Serve with 3 cups mixed baby greens tossed with a splash of balsamic vinegar.

Per serving: 400 calories, 21 g protein, 49 g carbohydrates, 15 g total fat, 3.5 g saturated fat, 11 g fiber, 396 mg sodium, 1,162 mg potassium

Kickstart | Day 5

Breakfast

Egg Melt and Fruit

Toast a slice of whole wheat bread, fold in half, and fill with 2 tablespoons shredded 2% reduced-fat Cheddar cheese, and 2 egg whites, scrambled. (On the go, have the Subway Egg White & Cheese Muffin Melt.) Have either option with 1 cup fat-free milk and 1 cup fresh or frozen and thawed unsweetened raspberries.

Breakaway Breakfast Option:

Have the raspberries.

Per serving: 280 calories, 21 g protein, 43 g carbohydrates, 2 g total fat, 1 g saturated fat, 8 g fiber, 595 mg sodium, 636 mg potassium

Lunch

Fast Frozen Meal

Have 1 Healthy Choice Complete Meals Beef Bourbon Dijon or Beef Tips Portobello with 1 multigrain flatbread-style cracker (Wasa brand or similar with about 45 calories each).

Per serving: 315–325 calories, 20–22 g protein, 43–44 g carbohydrates, 6–7 g total fat, 2–2.5 g saturated fat, 8 g fiber, 600–680 mg sodium, 630–700 mg potassium

Snack

Yogurt with Dates

Have ¾ cup 0% Greek yogurt and 5 dates.

Per serving: 200 calories, 16 g protein, 36 g carbohydrates, 1 g total fat, 0 g saturated fat, 3 g fiber, 60 mg sodium, 272 mg potassium

Dinner

Baked Potato, Turkey Breast, and Romaine Salad

Preheat the oven to 300°F. Whisk together 2 tablespoons rice vinegar, ½ teaspoon Dijon mustard, and ½ teaspoon dried rosemary. Pour into a resealable plastic bag. Add 3 ounces turkey breast tenderloin to the bag and marinate for at least 20 minutes. Pierce a large baking potato several times with a fork, rub the skin with ½ teaspoon olive oil, and place on a piece of foil. Bake for 1 hour 20 minutes to 1½ hours, or until slightly soft and golden brown. Top the potato with 2 tablespoons no-salt-added cottage cheese and 2 teaspoons chopped chives. Coat a saucepan with cooking spray and heat over medium-low heat. Cook the turkey for 3 minutes on each side, or until cooked through. Toss 2 cups romaine lettuce with a splash of balsamic vinegar.

Per serving: 400 calories, 32 g protein, 65 g carbohydrates, 2 g total fat, 0 g saturated fat, 11 g fiber, 150 mg sodium, 1,785 mg potassium

Kickstart | Day 6

Breakfast

Kiwifruit Yogurt Smoothie

In a blender, combine 1 cup fat-free plain yogurt, 4 small sliced kiwifruit, 2 tablespoons orange juice, and ½ teaspoon vanilla extract.

Breakaway Breakfast Option:

Make the smoothie and drink about one-third of it.
Save the rest for after your workout.

Per serving: 319 calories, 17 g protein, 61 g carbohydrates, 1 g total fat, 0 g saturated fat, 8 g fiber, 197 mg sodium, 1,520 mg potassium

Lunch

Balsamic Raisins and Tuna

Toss 3 tablespoons raisins with 2 tablespoons balsamic vinegar and ½ teaspoon olive oil. Stir together with 3 ounces low-sodium chunk light tuna packed in water, drained. Serve over 3 cups baby spinach. Serve with 1 cup fresh or unsweetened frozen and thawed raspberries.

Per serving: 296 calories, 26 g protein, 43 g carbohydrates, 4 g total fat, 0.5 g saturated fat, 11 g fiber, 210 mg sodium, 1,056 mg potassium

Snack

Roast Beef Crackers and Grapes

Have 1 multigrain flatbread-style cracker (such as Wasa) with 2 ounces low-sodium sliced roast beef (such as Applegate Farms) with ½ cup grapes.

Per serving: 177 calories, 15 g protein, 22 g carbohydrates, 3 g total fat, 1 g saturated fat, 3 g fiber, 280 mg sodium, 144 mg potassium

Dinner

Corn, Tomato, and Avocado Salad with "Chicken" Patty

Toss 1 cup cooked (from frozen) corn with 1 medium diced tomato and one-quarter avocado, chopped, with 2 tablespoons white vinegar, 1 teaspoon olive oil, and ½ teaspoon dried basil. Serve with 1 meat-free "chicken" patty (such as Morningstar Farms Chik Patties).

Per serving: 411 calories, 15 g protein, 56 g carbohydrates, 17 g total fat, 2.5 g saturated fat, 10 g fiber, 552 mg sodium, 1,077 mg potassium

Kickstart | Day 7

Breakfast

Cereal and Milk

Have 1½ cups Kellogg's Special K Protein Plus or Kashi GoLean with ¾ cup fat-free milk and one-quarter thinly sliced medium banana (save the rest of the banana for today's snack).

Breakaway Breakfast Option:

Have ½ cup of the cereal with ¼ cup fat-free milk.

Per serving: 289 calories, 27 g protein, 44 g carbohydrates, 6 g total fat, 1 g saturated fat, 11 g fiber, 297 mg sodium, 1,032 mg potassium

Lunch

Hearty Ham Pita

Stuff an 8-inch whole wheat pita (about 170 calories) with 2 ounces low-sodium ham (such as Applegate Farms), 1½ cups mixed baby greens, ¼ cup no-salt-added canned chickpeas, and a drizzle of white vinegar.

Per serving: 309 calories, 21 g protein, 51 g carbohydrates, 4 g total fat, 1 g saturated fat, 8 g fiber, 834 mg sodium, 413 mg potassium

Snack

Greek Yogurt with Pecans and Banana

Have 1 cup 0% Greek yogurt with three-quarters sliced medium banana (left over from breakfast) and 1 teaspoon pecans.

Per serving: 202 calories, 19 g protein, 29 g carbohydrates, 2 g total fat, 0 g saturated fat, 3 g fiber, 75 mg sodium, 326 mg potassium

Dinner

Vegetarian Chili

Have 1¾ cups low-sodium vegetarian chili (such as Health Valley Organic No Salt Added Tame Tomato Chili) with ½ ounce 2% reduced-fat shredded Cheddar cheese melted over the top.

Per serving: 408 calories, 21 g protein, 72 g carbohydrates, 7 g total fat, 2 g saturated fat, 14 g fiber, 243 mg sodium, 1,178 mg potassium

Common Questions about the Kickstart

Q Can I drink coffee on this plan?

A Feel free to include coffee or tea if you normally do so, but don't include this toward your goal of 64 ounces of water per day. Also, watch your calories for add-ons such as creamer and sugar. One tablespoon of fat-free creamer has about 10 calories, while 1 teaspoon of sugar has 16, and 1 teaspoon of honey has about 20. Make sure you choose a creamer without any partially hydrogenated oils.

Q What if I don't like a meal? Can I mix and match?

A For the Kickstart, it's best to keep the plan as intact as you can. (It's just 1 week, after all!) Each daily menu is carefully calibrated to balance the amounts of potassium and sodium, dietary minerals called electrolytes that help to balance the amount of water your body retains. Because a key part of the Kickstart is flushing out bloating, it's easiest to follow the registered dietitian–developed plan. However, if you are allergic to an ingredient in one meal (or simply don't like it), you can always skip that meal and eat one of the other meals on the plan twice. Just keep an eye on the potassium and sodium amounts in your other meals for the day to make sure the totals fall within the guidelines on page 140.

For the rest of the plan (beginning in the next chapter), it's fine to mix and match the different breakfasts, lunches, snacks, and dinners at will, and even make up your own meals, keeping the calorie, protein, fiber, and sodium guidelines in mind. The build-your-own-meal section starting on page 197 offers a quick reference guide to the nutrition facts of many foods you may want to incorporate.

Q. Eight cups sounds like a lot of water to drink. Any way to make it more interesting?

A. If you're not used to drinking the amount of water on this plan, 64 ounces of plain H_2O can seem like a lot. Tracy Gensler, RD, who developed the menus and nutrition guidelines for this plan, suggests the following low- or no-calorie twists on ordinary water to add a little taste to what comes out of your tap.

- **Citrus Refresher:** Add a lemon, lime, or orange wedge.
- **Juicy Water:** Add 1 to 2 tablespoons pomegranate, grape, orange, or cranberry juice to 16 ounces of water; just a little splash of juice adds big flavor.
- **Cool Green Tea:** Brew a cup of green tea and add 1 cup of cool water. Refrigerate and enjoy your tea cold.
- **Peppermint Burst:** Add a sprig of peppermint leaves.
- **Watermelon Cooler:** Puree some watermelon in your food processor, pour into ice cube trays, freeze, and add 1 cube to your water glass for a refreshing burst of flavor.

Q. There were fresh berries on sale at the grocery store this week. Can I substitute these for the frozen ones in the meal plan?

A. Absolutely. Fresh and frozen produce (fruits *and* veggies) are completely interchangeable in this plan as long as there's no added salt or sugar (check the label on the frozen variety to make sure the only ingredient is berries, for example).

Q I'm lactose intolerant. What can I have instead of the milk on this plan?

A In place of 1 cup of milk, you can swap in 1¼ cups light soy milk (10 ounces) or an identical amount of lactose-free milk for the same nutritional value. If you have a dairy allergy like one of our testers did (or are allergic to some other food on the plan), simply skip those meals and choose another option.

Q I usually drink a glass of wine with dinner. Can I drink alcohol on this plan?

A For a few reasons, it's best to avoid wine (and all alcohol), especially during this Kickstart week. The most obvious reason is that red wine consists of about 25 empty calories per ounce, which add to your daily tally without contributing any of the vitamins, minerals, or other nutrients you need. The second is that some studies have suggested that the relaxing effect of alcohol can cause people to lower their guard and eat more than they otherwise would. And finally, for the Kickstart (where one of the main goals is to reduce bloating), alcohol can actually irritate the stomach lining, making it harder to digest your dinner and actually contributing to excess bloating.

If your goal is to lose weight, the less alcohol—not to mention soda and other caloric beverages—you drink over the course of the program, the better. But that doesn't mean you have to be a teetotaler to succeed on this plan. In fact, plenty of glasses of wine found their way onto our test panelists' food logs. Just make sure you take stock of that roughly 100 calories per drink (not counting sugary mixers) and make it an occasional treat rather than a daily indulgence.

GET IN THE KNOW ABOUT
FROZEN MEALS

Frozen meals have come a long way from the days of the Hungry-Man fried chicken "TV dinner." With so many healthy (and tasty) options on the market, the freezer aisle can be a great option when cooking isn't in the cards. But calories and fat don't tell the whole story. Beware of meals that pack in excessive sodium or scrimp on fiber. Your nutrition goals for a dinner on this plan include 400 calories, at least 8 grams of fiber, no more than 4 grams of saturated fat, and at least 20 grams of protein. (After the Kickstart, the same will be true for lunch.) If you can find a frozen meal that fits into these guidelines, great! If not, when selecting frozen dinners, look for the following nutrition parameters:

○ At least 300 calories

○ No more than 4 grams of saturated fat

○ No more than 600 milligrams of sodium

○ At least 6 grams of fiber

○ At least 16 grams of protein

Add whole wheat flatbread-style crackers (such as Wasa) or slivered almonds to supplement fiber, calories, and protein. And round it out with frozen or fresh veggies.

Colleen Barnes

Age 47

Lost: 10 percent body fat

Gained: 14 percent increase in her upper-body strength

Favorite body part: Sculpted arms

Favorite exercise: Skater Side Twist. "It was tricky at first, but it uses so many muscles once you get the hang of it that I really came to love that one."

After gradually losing 10 pounds over the course of the last year through a combination of walking and healthier eating, Colleen Barnes, 47, was ready to focus on toning and strengthening. "I had zero upper-body strength," she says. Sitting in front of a computer screen all day left her shoulders and neck tight and knotted and her arms feeling weak and fatigued—so much so that something as seemingly simple as stirring up a batch of cookie dough required stopping to take a breather midway through. Not anymore. "I feel like I have so much more strength to do stuff than I did before."

Colleen had never done much strength training, but she was a fast fan of the bands. "If you're just using a dumbbell by itself, it's easy to be lax about it. But if you have resistance from the band, it keeps your focus right where it's supposed to be," she explains. Not to mention the portability: Even a spring break trip to Costa Rica with her stepdaughter's school travel club didn't derail her workouts, thanks to the ease of tossing the bands into her suitcase.

Exercise had always been an energizer for Colleen, but strength training turned out to have an added bonus: better sleep. Usually a very light sleeper, after strength workouts she slept more soundly and straight through the night.

Cutting back on salt also provided another unexpected lift. "I find that when I have salt, my calves swell," she says. "Without it, I feel so much more comfortable in my skin and clothes, and I have so much more energy and ability to move." While allergies to dairy and soy limited Colleen's food choices, she was still able to find some new favorites (and even some her husband would eat too!). Balsamic Raisins and Tuna (page 156) is now one of her go-to lunches.

"It's such a motivator to see and feel the differences in my body," says Colleen, raving about noticeable toning from her arms and upper chest to her hips and thighs (even after her prior weight loss, she managed to carve another inch each from her chest, waist, and thighs). "I've been out shopping because my clothes don't fit me anymore. I couldn't believe I bought a summer dress that was a size 4, and another sundress that was an extra small. I've never bought anything in extra small!"

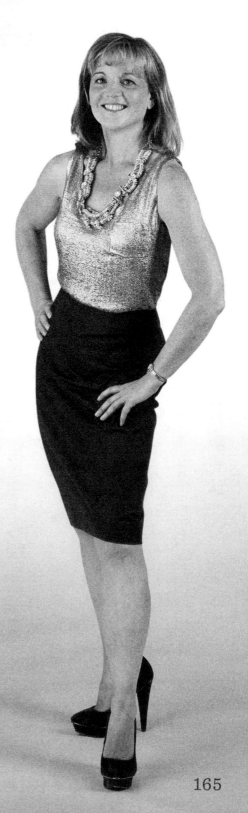

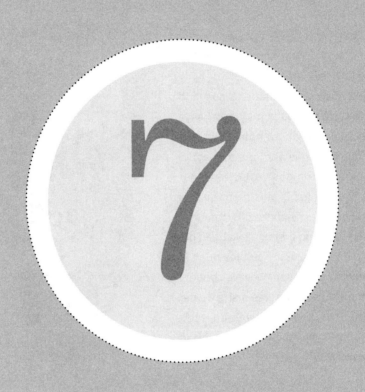

The 8-Week Tone Every Inch Program

Now that you've been introduced to the cardio and strength workouts that make up this plan, plus the 7-Day Kickstart diet, it's time to put the pieces together. The 8-Week Tone Every Inch Program is easiest to follow if you break it down into the 1-week Kickstart followed by three different phases in which we gradually increase the intensity of your workouts.

In each phase, you'll have a certain number of strength workouts (including different numbers of sets to aim for per workout) and cardio workouts (broken into Intensity and Moderate) to complete. Beyond those basic specifications, you can design your week in workouts however you like (see tips and a sample schedule on page 170).

The Phases

As I talked about in the beginning of the book, this workout program is grounded in the crucial concept of *progression* in exercise. Each phase is designed to build upon the last, allowing you to get the best results out of this plan without frustration, injury, or hitting those dreaded plateaus. Here's how it all breaks down.

The Kickstart

Week 1

- **Strength:** Do one or two sets of the band workout two times this week.
- **Cardio:** Do at least 20 minutes of Moderate Cardio two or three times this week.
- **Diet:** Follow the Kickstart nutrition plan in Chapter 6.

Think of the Kickstart as your initiation to the Tone Every Inch plan. The Kickstart diet in Chapter 6 is designed to rid your body of extra water weight and give you fast, motivating results that will propel you onward in the program.

The workouts are similarly designed to keep motivation high. While you may feel sore after these first strength workouts (especially if you haven't done any resistance exercise in a while!), the emphasis is on learning the moves—not slaving for hours in the gym.

Your goal for cardio this week is simply to get moving for 20 minutes two or three times. These Moderate Cardio sessions can be made up of anything you like to do: a brisk walk around the block a few times, a game of tennis with your husband—the choice is yours.

Phase I

Weeks 2 and 3

○ **Strength:** Do two or three sets of the band workout two times each week.

○ **Cardio:** Do two or three cardio workouts, including one Intensity Cardio workout.

○ **Diet:** Follow the Eating for Energy nutrition guidelines in Chapter 8.

By the second week of the program, you should have a good handle on the exercises and will (we hope) be doing less reading and more reps during your workouts! Our testers found that, while the first couple of times through it took upward of ½ hour or more to get through one set of all the exercises, once they got into the swing of things, they were able to knock out two sets in about 30 minutes.

Now that the strength routine is old hat, in Week 2 you'll add your first Intensity Cardio workout, as well as boost your Moderate Cardio workouts to a goal of 30 minutes.

Phase II

Weeks 4 and 5

○ **Strength:** Do one or two sets of the Triple-Toning workout twice in Week 4 and two or three sets twice in Week 5.

○ **Cardio:** Do two or three cardio workouts, including two Intensity Cardio workouts.

○ **Diet:** Follow the Eating for Energy nutrition guidelines in Chapter 8. Add a second snack if needed.

After 3 weeks of the band workout, it's time to up the ante and add some dumbbells as you do two Triple-Toning workouts this week. You are stronger than when you started the program, but it's still okay if you need to decrease the resistance of your band to do the exercises successfully with dumbbells, too. Get advice on finding the right combo in Chapter 4. Also, now that the moves have become a bit more complex—and a bit more challenging—it's a good idea to back it off for a week while you get used to the new moves. That's why I suggest doing just one or two sets in Week 4 before bumping it back up to two or three sets in Week 5.

In the cardio department, keep on inching up the proportion of your workouts that are Intensity Cardio as you get both stronger and fitter. Bump it up to two Intensity Cardio workouts in this phase of the program.

Phase III

Weeks 6 to 8

- ○ **Strength:** Do two or three sets of the Triple-Toning workout two or three times each week.
- ○ **Cardio:** Do two or three Intensity Cardio workouts. Moderate Cardio is optional during this phase.
- ○ **Diet:** Follow the Eating for Energy nutrition guidelines in Chapter 8. Add a second snack if needed.

You've hit the home stretch! At this stage you can add an optional third strength workout if you like. If you're feeling good, you can also try the "Make It Harder" versions of the exercises in Chapter 4.

For cardio, it's all about intensity. In this final phase, do up to three Intensity Cardio workouts. You don't need to do any Moderate Cardio unless you want to.

Sample 8-Week Schedule

The following calendar shows different ways you can customize the program to fit your schedule. The only hard-and-fast rule is to never do two strength workouts or two Intensity Cardio workouts on back-to-back days. That's because in order to change your body, you have to actually damage your muscles (in a good way!) so they heal stronger than before (more on that in Chapter 9). But the key to realizing the body-toning benefits of the workouts you're doing is to give your muscles time to recuperate by doing something different the day after a hard workout. You may think that rest is best when you're feeling sore, but a rest day isn't always called for. Doing some Moderate Cardio— enough to get your blood pumping without being super-strenuous— can actually help to reduce soreness because the increased bloodflow carries important healing nutrients to your muscles, helping them to feel better faster. Following a Moderate Cardio session with some gentle stretching is a great idea. The routine on page 180 will get you started.

One of the easiest ways to adapt the workout plan to fit your schedule is to choose whether you'd rather do workouts most days of a week and limit them to no more than 30 minutes a day, or if you'd rather double up, doing cardio and strength workouts in the same day, which will give you a longer workout session but a bonus day off.

The pieces of the puzzle:

○ **Strength workouts:** For the Kickstart plus Phase I (Weeks 1 through 3), these will be band-only workouts, then for Phases II and III (Weeks 4 through 8), they will be combo (band/dumbbell) workouts.

○ **Intensity Cardio workouts:** Starting with Phase I (Weeks 2 and 3), you'll add one Intensity Cardio workout. In Phase II (Weeks 4 and 5), you'll add a second interval workout, and in Phase III (Weeks 6 through 8), you'll have the option of adding a third.

○ **Moderate Cardio workouts:** You'll begin with just a couple of 20-minute sessions (doing virtually any activity you like that doesn't involve weights) during the Kickstart (Week 1). In Phases I and II (Weeks 2 through 5), you'll bump those workouts up in length, aiming for 30 minutes. In Phase III (Weeks 6 through 8), these workouts are optional so you can do as much or as little as feels good.

Sample 8-Week Calendar

	MONDAY	TUESDAY	WEDNESDAY	
Kickstart				
Week 1	Band workout: 1 set	20-min elliptical	Day off	
Phase I				
Week 2	Fat Blast Minute Intervals	Band workout: 2 sets	Day off	
Week 3	Band workout: 2 sets	Day off	30-min stationary bike	
Phase II				
Week 4	Combo strength workout: 1 set	Fat Blast Minute Intervals	Zumba class (30 min) (optional)	
Week 5	Combo strength workout: 2 sets	25-min treadmill walk/jog (optional)	Fat Blast 30-Second Intervals	
Phase III				
Week 6	Combo strength workout: 3 sets + Fat Blast 30-Second Intervals	15-min walk (optional)	Combo strength workout: 2 sets + Fat Blast Minute Intervals	
Week 7	Combo strength workout: 3 sets	Fat Blast 30-Second Intervals	Combo strength workout: 2 sets + 30-min stair machine (optional)	
Week 8	Combo strength workout: 3 sets	Day off	Combo strength workout: 2 sets + Fat Blast 30-Second Intervals	

Dress for Fitness Success

Don't worry, you don't have to go out and spend lots of money on a new workout wardrobe to do this program. But a few key pieces can make your workouts feel better—and make you feel more confident doing them.

THURSDAY	FRIDAY	SATURDAY	SUNDAY
Band workout: 1 set	Day off	20-min walk	20-min bike ride (optional)
Band workout: 2 sets + 30-min walk	Day off	Step aerobics DVD (optional)	Day off
Band workout: 2 sets	Day off	Fat Blast 30-Second Intervals	20-min elliptical (optional)
Combo strength workout: 2 sets	Water aerobics (45 min) (optional)	Fat Blast Minute Intervals	Day off
Day off	Combo strength workout: 2 sets	Day off	Fat Blast Minute Intervals
Day off	Combo strength workout: 3 sets (optional)	Day off	Roller skating (30 min) (optional)
Fat Blast Minute Intervals	Combo strength workout: 3 sets (optional)	Day off	20-Minute Power Blast (at local 5-K) (optional)
Walk with a friend (optional)	Combo strength workout: 3 sets	Fat Blast Minute Intervals	Nature hike (1 hr) (optional)

Shoes. This is the one place you might have to spend some money if you don't already own a pair of comfortable athletic shoes. But they don't have to break the bank. In fact, the most expensive sneakers you can buy probably aren't any better than versions that cost half as much, if you ask a group of researchers from the University of Dundee in Scotland who put running shoes at three different price points to the test. They measured both the amount of pressure on different parts of the bottom of the foot (a gauge of how well the cushioning worked) as well as the wearers' comfort ratings. No connection was found between price and cushioning or feel-good factor.

If you run, shoes made for running are a must. As a walker, running or walking shoes will do the trick. If you like to mix it up (or you haven't decided yet), walking or running shoes are generally a safe bet, or you might try what's called a cross trainer, or a multipurpose exercise shoe. Some cross trainers are designed to offer lateral, or side-to-side sup-

THE TONE EVERY INCH EXPRESS

If you feel, as did several of our test panelists, that spending 30 minutes a day on a workout feels either incredibly boring or like a challenging amount of time to find in one chunk, this express modification of the routine breaks down the strength exercises from Chapters 3 and 4 into two shorter routines you can do on back-to-back days. One caveat: Because many of the exercises in this program target upper- and lower-body muscles simultaneously, it's impossible to break the routine into exclusive upper- and lower-body moves, which would be ideal for this type of back-to-back training. (In other words, there will be some overlap where similar muscles will be involved in both workouts, so listen to your body.) If a particular muscle is feeling extra sore, take a day off from strength altogether.

Express workout 1:

1. Cheerleader Press

2. Two-Way Row

3. Pullover and Crunch

4. Chest Press

5. Side Leg-Lift Crunch

Express workout 2:

1. Pickup and Shrug

2. Lunge Repeater

3. Skater Side Twist

4. Butt Kicker

5. Squat and Curl

port, which can be helpful for workouts that involve moving in all different directions (like cardio dance or step classes), as opposed to the straightforward motion of walking, running, and most cardio machines. While buying online is often cheaper, if this is the first athletic shoe purchase you've made in a while, I recommend making it an in-person buy. A reputable sporting goods or specialty running store will have salespeople who are trained to fit you to the right shoe size (even if you've worn the same size for years, you might be surprised). Plus you'll want to walk or jog around in the shoe to make sure it feels good right out of the box (don't count on "breaking in" an initially uncomfortable shoe). If you do go the online route, take care to buy from a merchant with a generous return policy and wear the shoes indoors on carpet before you commit.

Clothing. Sure, a ratty old college sweatshirt and sweatpants are perfectly adequate dress for these workouts. As long as you can move comfortably, you're good to go. But let me tell you something: Exercise clothing has come a long way, baby. While cotton used to be the go-to fabric for getting active, fabrics have gotten a lot smarter. Here are some features to look for if you decide to invest in some new pieces.

○ *Tag says:* Wicking
   What it means: While cotton tends to soak up sweat and hang on to it, newer "technical" fabrics (like CoolMax or Dri-FIT) are designed with fibers that actually work to pull moisture away from your body and allow it to evaporate more quickly from the outside of the garment so you stay cooler when it's hot and warmer when it's cold. Drier clothing—from shirts to undergarments to socks—means less rubbing.

○ *Tag says:* Antimicrobial
   What it means: Whereas early technical fabrics were prone to smelliness, now many fabrics are given germ-killing treatments that include weaving in silver fibers or even material from recycled coconut shells, both of which have inherent antistink properties. (Germs are what cause sweat to smell.)

SHOULD I GO BAREFOOT?

Virtually since athletic shoes came to be, shoe manufacturers have been competing to see who can add the most bells and whistles, pack in the most foot-cradling cushioning, and engineer the best support system for the foot.

But in recent years there's been a shift toward a less-is-more mentality, with the extreme being exercisers who go so far as to run marathons completely barefoot, or in Vibram FiveFingers, shoes that are little more than rubber gloves for the feet to protect them from things like broken glass. On the less extreme end of things, most major shoe manufacturers now offer styles that bring your foot closer to barefoot by providing less cushion and support.

The argument for giving up your cushiest kicks is that all of that padding provides you with a false sense of security, encouraging you to pound your feet harder than you would if you were barefoot. For example, some studies have shown that runners wearing traditional running shoes land on their heels, which creates 30 percent greater shock to the knees than runners in "minimalist" shoes made to mimic being barefoot, who landed on the middle or front of their feet and managed to spread out the impact.

Experts who like barefoot running argue that wearing shoes is like wearing a neck brace to hold your head up—eventually the muscles underneath would wither away so you wouldn't be able to hold your head up on your own anymore. For your feet, advocates say, taking away the support of traditional footwear means the muscles in your feet will have to work harder and as a result will grow stronger and able to better support themselves.

When I asked Reed Ferber, PhD, assistant professor of kinesiology and director of the Running Injury Clinic at the University of Calgary in Canada, he told me that about 80 percent of people have healthy enough feet to wear shoes with less support (the rest are outliers with either extremely flexible or extremely rigid arches that are better off with more structured shoes). But if you are going to try them, it's important to treat wearing them like a new workout, he warns. Build up slowly, starting with no more than 10 percent of your total exercise time in them, and gradually increasing it by about 10 percent a week.

○ *Tag says:* UPF

What it means: Think of it as SPF for your clothes. Whether or not you've ever noticed the rays seeping through your clothing, that white cotton T-shirt only gets a UPF score of 5, meaning that one-fifth, or 20 percent, of the damaging UVA and UVB rays make it through. A thicker weave and darker color help—blue jeans come in at a UPF 50+—but they're not very comfortable for working out. Luckily, these days many sportswear makers offer cool, light-weight fabrics with UPF values of up to 50+ that protect your skin while keeping you cool.

A sports watch. In this day of constantly attached cell phones that do everything from keep your calendar to make your grocery lists, wristwatches seem to be falling out of fashion. But while many phones do have a stopwatch function, I find it easier to use a good old-fashioned watch to track my interval workouts. You can get one with basic chronograph function (that's watch lingo for being able to track both the time of day and the duration of your workout) for as little as $10. For around $30 and up you can find watches that allow you to program in your interval splits (for example, have it beep every 30 seconds or every minute so you can speed up and slow down on cue).

The Importance of Staying Flexible

Whether or not you played on a sports team as a child, you probably had gym class of some sort. And before you got on with whatever game was on the agenda for the day, the teacher probably led the class through some basic stretches. This pre-exercise ritual has been ingrained in our culture for decades, but in recent years there's been a lot of debate among the scientific community about whether we've stretched (sorry!) our expectations. In fact, some scientists have even reported that stretching might temporarily *decrease* measures of physical performance such as strength, speed, and power (a combo of the first two). Other scientists point out the flaws in that research, claiming that those findings don't apply in real life.

While studies are certainly ongoing, a trio of researchers with the Centers for Disease Control and Prevention reviewed 361 different studies spanning nearly 40 years to come up with some conclusions based on the best information we have. Their investigation determined that preworkout stretching won't keep you from getting sore, and it has not been shown to do much for your injury risk. However, there are still plenty of reasons to get your stretch on. Here are a few.

Stretch for heart health. You hardly think of your inability to touch your toes as a sign of increased heart disease risk, but several studies suggest that might just be the case. In fact, adults who were able to reach at least 12 inches past their toes (picture the sit-and-reach test from gym class) had 30 percent less stiffening of the arteries than less limber peers. More pliable arteries have an easier time expanding and contracting as blood pumps through, spelling lower blood pressure.

It feels good. Okay, so remember how I said stretching couldn't prevent (or heal) muscle soreness? Well, that's still true, but there is a little something stretching *can* do for sore, tight, or otherwise overworked muscles: It can make them feel better. A contradiction, you say? Not exactly. Time is still the only way to heal muscle soreness for good, but that blissfully relaxed sensation that you feel when you *streeetch* is capable of making you feel better—temporarily. Just don't stretch too aggressively or you risk further damage to your sore muscles.

Improve your posture. Imagine the way many elderly people walk—hunched over and shuffling with partially bent knees. If you spend your days sitting at a desk hunched over a computer, that might just be where you're headed. That's because spending hours a day seated without doing any flexibility exercises to counteract it can leave you with very tight hip and chest muscles. Hips get tight because they're hanging out in a shortened (flexed) position for as long as you're sitting (an average of 7.7 hours a day). Over time, they can become so tight that it's difficult to stand up straight. As for the chest and shoulders, hunching over your computer (or steering wheel) freezes those muscles in a compromised position, gradually shortening their length.

Avoid injury. I know, I just told you stretching didn't prevent injuries. And it doesn't—if you just stretch once, that is. An inflexible person is still more likely to pull a muscle than a flexible person, though—you just have to stretch regularly over time to benefit. And here's some good news: It turns out that we aren't doomed to lose flexibility as we get older, according to Michael Bemben, PhD, professor and chair of the department of health and exercise science at the University of Oklahoma in Norman. Rather, the loss of flexibility happens when we don't use the range of motion we have. Just 10 to 15 minutes of stretching three times a week can help you to turn the corner, though—even if you'll never be able to touch your toes.

How to Do It

When you stretch a muscle, you're actually stretching the connective tissue (including tendons and ligaments) that surrounds the muscles and bones, holding everything together.

Warm up first. You don't have to do your stretching in conjunction with a workout, but you will get more lasting lengthening if your muscles aren't stone cold. An increase of just 1 to 3 degrees above normal is enough to make a difference. If you don't have time at the end of your strength or cardio workouts to fit in stretching, try it after a warm shower (or while you suds up).

Aim for at least three sessions a week. Whether you stretch postworkout as a part of your cooldown when your muscles are toasty, or in the evening during your favorite TV show, the benefits of stretching require regular practice. And like so many elements of exercise, stretching is a use-it-or-lose-it game. It takes about 6 weeks for the increase in flexibility to stick, but even after that, if you stop stretching, your body will return to its prior inflexible self.

Hold it! Pulling and bouncing does not a loose muscle make. In fact, it's quite the opposite. If you try to throw yourself into the splits (without sufficient flexibility to do so), your body has a handy trick up its sleeve. If you try to stretch too far too fast, a team of sensory organs sends a message to the muscle, telling it to quickly contract, stopping the stretch in its tracks. Slow, gradual stretching, on the other hand, increases the length of time that the muscle will stay lengthened. Hold each stretch for 15 to 30 seconds.

Stretches to Try

These moves will help you loosen up the seven muscle groups most affected by your new cardio and strength-training routines. Just follow the directions for each number to get the maximum stretch from head to toe.

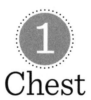

Chest

(most likely to feel tight from: Chest Press)

Stand facing an open doorway with your feet about hip-width apart. Open your arms out to the sides, elbows bent, and place one hand on either side of the door frame at shoulder height. Hinge forward from your ankles, leaning into the door until you feel a gentle stretch.

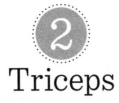

Triceps

(most likely to feel tight from: Cheerleader Press and Pullover and Crunch)

Reach your right arm overhead next to your ear, then bend at the elbow as though you're going to scratch your shoulder blade. Reach your left hand across to grasp the right elbow, which is now sticking straight up. Gently press down with your left hand until you feel a stretch in the back of your right arm. Hold, then switch sides and do it again.

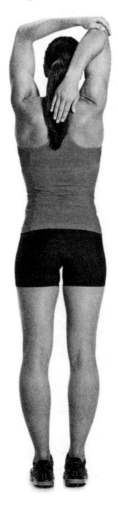

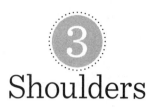

3
Shoulders

(most likely to feel tight from: Two-Way Row
and Cheerleader Press)

Reach your right arm across your body at about chest level. Place your left arm on your right upper arm and press it gently toward your body to feel a stretch in the back of your shoulder. Hold, then switch sides and do it again.

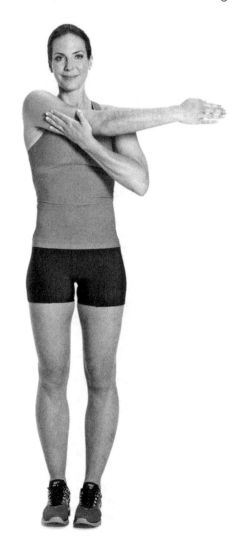

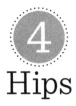

4

Hips

(most likely to feel tight from: Skater Side Twist and Lunge Repeater)

Get down on one knee. That's right, just like you're about to pop the question. Now shift your front knee forward until you feel a stretch in your back hip. Hold, then switch sides and do it again.

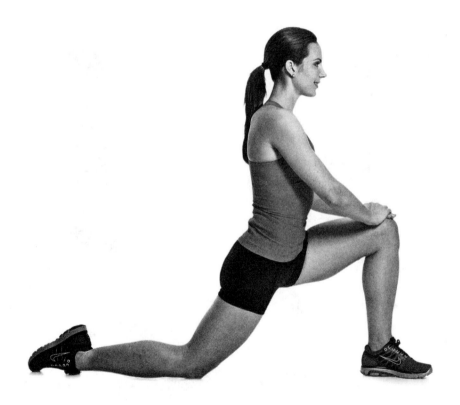

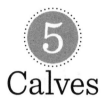

Calves

(most likely to feel tight from: Intensity Cardio workouts)

Standing with your feet hip-width apart, bend your left knee slightly and take a big step back with your right foot. With your right leg straight, press your right heel into the ground (Photo A) to feel a stretch in the back of your lower leg (slide your right foot back if needed until you feel the stretch). Hold the stretch, then bend your back knee slightly until you feel a stretch in your shin, or the front of the lower leg (Photo B). Hold that stretch, then switch sides and do it again.

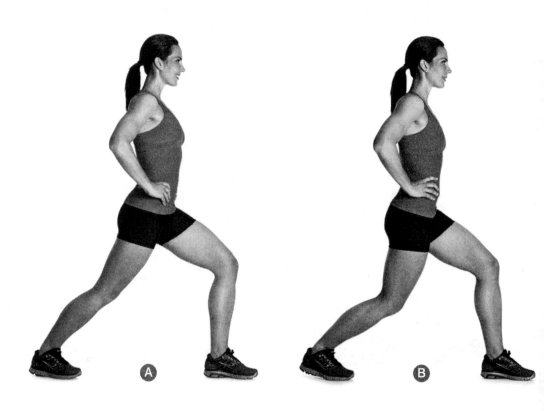

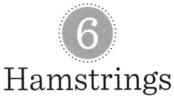

6
Hamstrings

(most likely to feel tight from: Butt Kicker and Squat and Curl)

There are two good ways to stretch this muscle, which runs down the back of your upper leg, just below your rear end. Take your pick, depending on whether you prefer to do it standing or lying down.

Standing hamstring stretch. Starting with your feet hip-width apart, pick up your right foot and place just the heel down about 12 inches in front of your left foot. Hinge your upper body forward from your hips, interlacing your fingers and pressing into your right thigh. You should feel a stretch in the back of your upper leg. Hold, then switch sides and do it again.

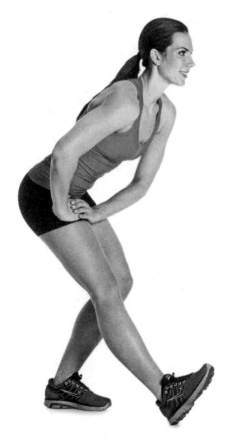

(continued)

Floor hamstring stretch. Lie on your back on a comfortable surface (an exercise mat or carpet works, or you can even do this one in bed or on a couch!). Bend your right knee, placing the foot flat on the floor, and grasp the back of your left upper leg with both hands. Gently pull your left leg toward your body, keeping the knee straight. Hold, then switch sides and do it again.

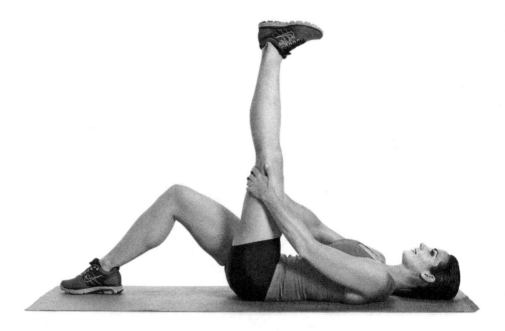

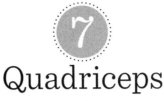

Quadriceps

(most likely to feel tight from: Squat and Curl and Lunge Repeater)

Stand with your feet shoulder-width apart, a sturdy chair or countertop within reach in case you need to hold onto something for balance. Reach back with your right hand to grab your right foot or ankle, bending at the knee. Make sure your hips are facing forward and your knees stay in line with each other as you gently press your heel toward your rear to feel a stretch in the front of your right thigh. Hold, then switch sides and do it again.

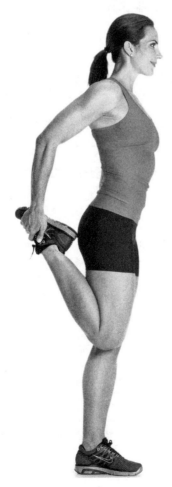

FINDING YOUR EQUILIBRIUM

Whether or not it's even on your radar, your balance—the ability to stay upright and steady—starts to gradually deteriorate as early as age 25. A number of factors are at play, and just by doing this program, you're on the right track. That's because strong muscles play a major role in whether you feel wobbly or sure-footed. But behind the large muscles of the arms, legs, and midsection that we focus on in this book, tiny stabilizer muscles are working together to keep you upright. Balance is also about strengthening neural pathways that help you to sense and react to things like a changing surface under your feet. If you are feeling unsteady as you do the exercises in this book, practicing some simple balance skills can help you get up to speed. Don't worry—this won't take much time, and it's a perfect thing to sneak in while you're waiting for the microwave, standing in line, or even brushing your teeth.

A note on safety: When you're starting out, make sure to try these exercises next to a countertop, chair, or wall that you can grab onto if you feel unsteady.

Level 1: Narrowing Base

Start by standing with your feet together, hands on your hips (Photo A). Can you stand like this for 30 seconds? If it's a challenge for you, stay here, and practice a couple times a day. If you're comfortable, move on to the next challenge.

Stand with your feet in a line, heel to toe, hands on your hips (Photo B). Can you stand like this for 30 seconds? If it's a challenge for you, stay here, and practice a couple times a day. If you're comfortable, move on to the next challenge.

Walk heel to toe in a straight line, hands at your sides. Can you walk across the room like this without difficulty? If it's a challenge for you, stay here and practice a couple times a day. If you're comfortable, move on to the next challenge.

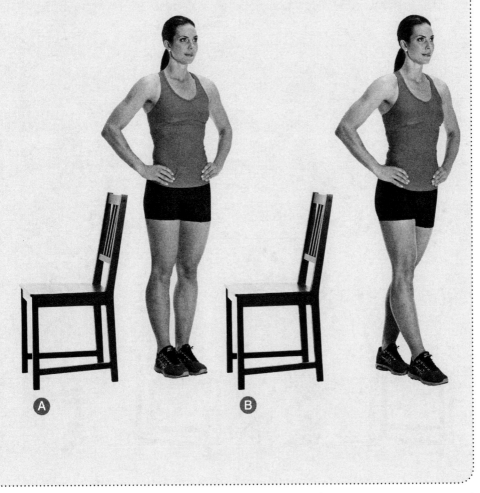

(continued)

FINDING YOUR EQUILIBRIUM (cont.)

Level 2: Mastering One-Foot Balance

Start with your feet hip-width apart. Pick up your right foot and hold it out to the front slightly (Photo A). Can you stand like this for 30 seconds? Repeat holding your leg to the side, then to the back. If it's a challenge for you, stay here, and practice a couple times a day on each leg. If you're comfortable, move on to the next challenge.

March in place in slow motion. Bring each knee up to hip level, pause in midair, then lower and repeat with the other side (Photo B).

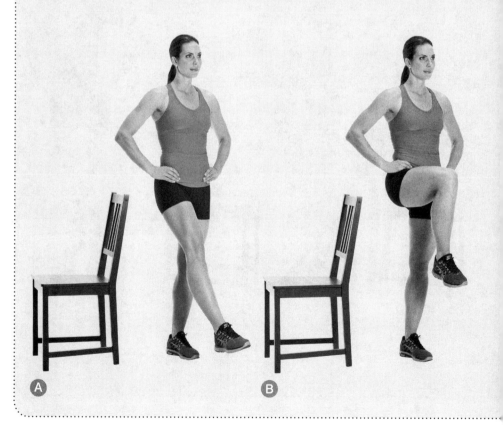

Level 3: Setting It in Motion

Standing on your right foot, lift your left foot straight to the front (Photo A). Hold for a count of 5, then bring it back to center. Lift your left leg to the side (Photo B), hold, then return to center. Repeat to the back, then return to center. For an extra challenge, don't touch the left foot down between each lift. Repeat on the other side, balancing on your left leg this time. Got it? Move on to the next challenge.

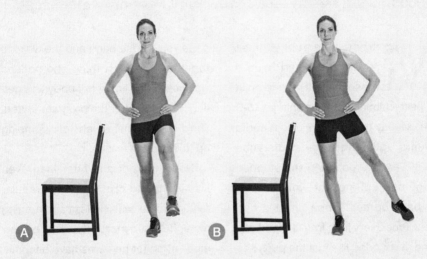

Stand next to a chair for balance if needed and stand on your left leg, right knee bent behind you. Bend your standing knee and hinge forward from your waist, reaching to touch the ground or as close as you can get without toppling (Photo C). Return to standing (but try not to touch down with your right foot). Work up to sets of 10 reps.

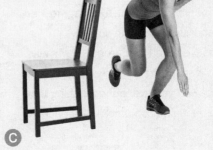

Lisa McCutcheon

Age 49

Lost: 6 pounds of fat and 7 percent body fat

Gained: 33 percent more leg strength

Favorite newly sculpted body part: "The whole area just under my bust. I can see my ribs again, and I have my waist back!"

Married to a runner, Lisa McCutcheon had been a runner herself off and on in the past, culminating in finishing a 15-K race (slightly more than 9 miles) about 5 years ago—the longest distance she'd ever covered. Then she stopped altogether, putting her workouts on the back burner. When she learned about Tone Every Inch from a friend of a friend, it sounded like just the push she needed.

Lisa never had to worry about her weight when she was younger. "But after children and after menopause, my metabolism came to a screeching halt," she says. She knew muscle tone was the magic ingredient to bringing her metabolism back up to speed.

Lisa doesn't sugarcoat it. "I was really sore in the first few weeks," she says. "But I've never done anything that gave me results so quickly—especially once you did the band and the weights together." The first thing she noticed was how much firmer her body was getting. A month after the program ended, she'd doubled her weight loss, jumping up to 8 pounds lost.

Now stronger and fitter than ever, Lisa is shaving minutes off her regular running route, walking less and running more. But she's most astounded by how much stronger her arms have become. "I remember that first day struggling to put that bar up," she says, describing the strength test. "It's not a struggle anymore, and I have so much more energy—even just doing chores.

"I can tell in clothing just how different a shape I am," she says. "My waist and my legs have always been my trouble spots. Now the waist area and my legs are so much firmer and thinner in clothing, and my arms are less jiggly." Now she can't wait to show it all off in tank tops and shorts—something she never would have felt comfortable wearing before. "I always hated shorts. I hadn't bought them in 3 years," Lisa says. "I just went out and bought two new pairs of Bermuda shorts. I was so self-conscious of my thighs and my back end and I'm not anymore. I was amazed at the size I fit into and that I liked how it looked! It was a fantastic feeling." Even her 19-year-old daughter couldn't believe the transformation when she came home from college, telling Lisa: "Mom, you look awesome."

The positive changes extend beyond Lisa's clothing options, too. "I forgot how good it felt to be in shape," she says. "So many of my friends have given up on working out, but what women don't realize is with all these changes in menopause—trouble with depression, mood swings, even sleep patterns get askew—really, that heavy-duty working out is what helps you." Stressful events in her personal life, including her father being hospitalized 3 hours away, could have completely derailed her progress. But instead, her workouts served as an island of sanity that helped her to stay calm and feel in control of something. "I'd forgotten how much of a stress release it is to work out," she says.

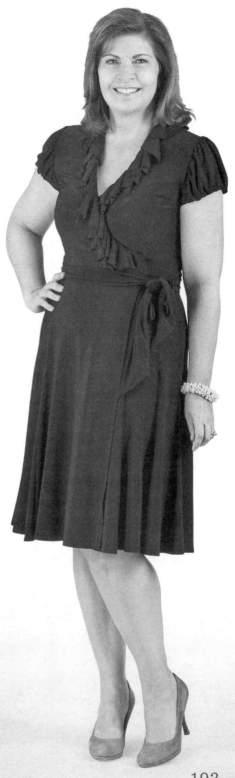

193

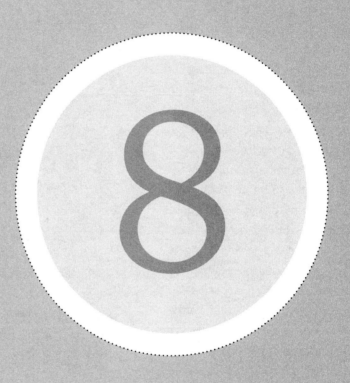

Eating for Energy— And Faster Firming

Unlike your run-of-the-mill weight loss diet plan, this program is about more than cutting calories. It's about getting proper nutrition—with plenty of protein to support metabolism-stoking muscle development— to energize and enhance the benefits of the workouts you're doing while supporting your weight loss goals. For tester Ann Warde, 54, who lost 3.5 pounds on the program, concentrating on getting enough protein made all the difference in her energy level—so much so that she found she doesn't need as much caffeine to help her power through the afternoon anymore. For tester Merry Buckley, the combination of protein and fiber helped her cut calories without going hungry. Like the exercise plan in this book, the eating plan also has progression built in. Quite simply, as your workouts pick up steam, you'll need to increase your calorie intake to make sure you're fully fueled. The first phase, also known as the Lighten-Up 7-Day Kickstart, was detailed in Chapter 6. This chapter begins with Week 2 and lays out the next 7 weeks of the program.

The Eating-for-Energy Principles

While the Kickstart diet plan was designed to keep calories low, increase your potassium, and limit your sodium intake in order to reduce bloating, we recommend following that plan only for the first week of the program. That's because the Kickstart diet won't give you quite enough calories to stay energized through longer and more intense workouts, and the last thing you want is to stunt your progress by eating too few calories.

Therefore, while some of the basic nutrition guidelines for Weeks 2 through 8 of the program are very similar to the Lighten-Up 7-Day Kickstart (the water, protein, fiber, and saturated fat recommendations remain the same), there are some changes as well. You'll increase your calorie goal from 1,200 to 1,400 a day, relax your sodium limit to 2,300 milligrams a day (the American Dietetic Association's recommended limit), and stop counting potassium. In addition, as your workouts get harder, you'll see that you have the option to add an additional 200 calories per day, for a total of 1,600. Here's the breakdown.

○ Each day, aim to eat three 400-calorie meals plus a 200-calorie snack, totaling 1,400 calories (if you're over 5-foot-8 or find yourself feeling hungry or sluggish, you might need to add a second snack, bumping your total to 1,600 calories).

○ You'll get 20 grams of protein from each meal and 15 grams from each snack to fuel muscle sculpting and help you feel satisfied.

○ You'll aim for a maximum of 2,300 milligrams of sodium per day.

○ You'll limit your saturated fat intake to no more than 10 percent of your calories (or no more than 14 grams; 16 if you've added the second snack).

○ Each meal will contain at least 8 grams of fiber.

○ You'll drink 8 cups (64 ounces) of water each day to help flush out toxins, carry nutrients to your cells, and prevent dehydration-triggered lethargy.

○ Each breakfast offers a "Breakaway Breakfast" option with about 15 grams of carbohydrate to allow you to munch something first thing if you plan to do an a.m. workout.

How to Create Tone Every Inch Meals

Prefer to start from scratch and create your own meal plan? Whether you're throwing together a turkey sandwich for lunch on the go, choosing ingredients from the salad bar, or just want to get creative at home, here's a quick reference guide to the nutrients essential to the Tone Every Inch diet. Pick any combination of foods that help you meet the goals below in the Tone Every Inch Food Formula. You can also use the information in this guide to substitute like foods for each other in the recipes and menus you'll find throughout this book; for example, trading an orange for an apple, or mixed baby greens for baby spinach. Later in this chapter you'll find almost 40 simple and delicious recipes that meet the guidelines.

Tone Every Inch Food Formula

Follow these guidelines to design your own meals that meet the recommended nutrition goals of the Tone Every Inch plan.

Daily Goals

75 grams of protein minimum

25 grams of fiber minimum

1,400 to 1,600 calories maximum

2,300 milligrams of sodium maximum

14 to 16 grams of saturated fat maximum

Step-by-Step Meals

1. Pick a protein source (goal: 20 grams of protein). *Note:* Because you'll pick up a few bonus grams of protein from other components of your meal, you'll only need to aim for about 15 grams of protein from your main protein source.

2. Add fiber-rich foods (goal: 8 grams of fiber). *Note:* Make sure to get a variety of fruits, vegetables, and grains throughout the day.

3. Account for any extras (total calorie goal: 400).

4. Total your protein, fiber, and calories to make sure you're meeting your goals. If not, adjust the portions as needed.

Step-by-Step Snacks

1. Pick a protein source (goal: 15 grams of protein). *Note:* Because you'll pick up a few bonus grams of protein from other components of your snack, you'll only need to aim for about 10 grams of protein from your main protein source.

2. Add fiber-rich foods (goal: 2 grams of fiber). *Note:* Make sure to get a variety of fruits, vegetables, and grains throughout the day.

3. Account for any extras (total calorie goal: 200).

4. Total your protein, fiber, and calories to make sure you're meeting your goals. If not, adjust the portions as needed.

Step 1: Choose a Lean Protein Source

For maximum muscle toning, aim for at least 20 grams of muscle-nourishing protein per 400-calorie meal and 15 grams per 200-calorie snack. But when you're choosing a protein component, remember that you don't have to get it all in one spot. That's because you can usually count on getting at least a few grams from the other foods you'll be incorporating (for example, a 100-calorie slice of whole wheat bread adds 5 grams of protein—not bad!). As a rule of thumb, try to get at least 15 grams from your main protein source (like meat, beans, tofu, dairy, etc.) for meals and at least 10 grams from snacks.

The calorie counts below do not include any fat used in preparation. If you use oil or butter, remember to account for the calories from fat in this chart.

Vegetarian Choices

FOOD	SERVING SIZE	CALORIES	PROTEIN	FIBER
Black beans, low sodium or no-salt-added	1¼ cups	250	18 g	21 g
Boca Original Vegan Burger*	1 patty	100	19 g	6 g
Cannellini beans, low sodium or no-salt-added	1¼ cups	200	15 g	14 g
Chickpeas, low sodium or no-salt-added	1¼ cups	250	15 g	9 g
Edamame, shelled	1 cup	244	17 g	8 g
Health Valley Organic No-Salt-Added Tomato Chili*	1 cup	315	15 g	12 g
Kidney beans, low sodium or no-salt-added	1 cup	220	16 g	14 g
Lentils, low sodium or no-salt-added	1 cup	200	16 g	16 g
Lentil soup, no-salt-added	1 cup	140	9 g	8 g
Minestrone soup, no-salt-added	1 cup	90	4 g	3 g
Morningstar Veggie Breakfast Sausage Patties*	2 patties	160	20 g	2 g
Special K Protein Plus Cereal*	1¼ cups	167	17 g	8 g
Tofu	7 oz	139	16 g	1.8 g

*The nutrition values for these foods will vary according to brand. Please use these values as a goal when selecting your product.

Meat, Fish, Egg, and Dairy Choices

FOOD	SERVING SIZE	CALORIES	PROTEIN	FIBER
Beef tenderloin, cooked	3 oz	135	18 g	0 g
Cheddar cheese, reduced fat	1 oz	91	7 g	0 g
Chicken breast, cooked	2 oz	94	18 g	0 g
Chunk light tuna, in water	3 oz	90	20 g	0 g
Cottage cheese, 1% fat	½ cup	81	14 g	0 g
Crabmeat, cooked	3 oz	74	15 g	0 g
Dark meat chicken, cooked	2 oz	116	16 g	0 g
Eggs	2 large	143	13 g	0 g
Egg whites	⅔ cup	78	18 g	0 g
Fat-free ricotta cheese	¾ cup	120	18 g	0 g
Greek yogurt, 0%	1 cup	100	16 g	0 g
Ground beef (95% lean), cooked	2 oz	97	15 g	0 g
Ham, deli sliced	3 oz	75	15 g	0 g
Mackerel, cooked	3 oz	174	16 g	0 g
Milk, fat-free	1½ cups	125	12 g	0 g
Mozzarella, reduced fat	1 oz	70	6 g	0 g
Pork tenderloin, cooked	2 oz	91	17 g	0 g
Roast beef, deli sliced	3 oz	120	18 g	0 g
Salmon, cooked	3 oz	120	17 g	0 g
Soy milk, fat-free	2 cups	140	12 g	1 g
Turkey breast, deli sliced	3 oz	75	18 g	0 g
Yogurt, fat-free, plain	1 cup (or 8 oz)	137	14 g	0 g
Yogurt, light, flavored	6 oz	100	6 g	0 g

Step 2: Choose Fiber-Rich Complements

Next, fill out your meal with a variety of fruits, vegetables, and/or whole grains. While there's no hard-and-fast rule about how many of each you must have in each meal, do make sure you get a variety of each over the course of the day, emphasizing fruits and veggies first. In the tables that follow, note that all fruits and vegetables are raw, unless otherwise specified.

Vegetables

FOOD	SERVING SIZE	CALORIES	PROTEIN	FIBER
Alfalfa sprouts	½ cup	4	0.7 g	0.3 g
Arugula	3 cups	15	1.5 g	2 g
Asparagus	5 medium spears	16	1.8 g	2 g
Bell pepper (any color)	½ cup, chopped	23	0.7 g	2 g
Broccoli	1 cup	31	3 g	2 g
Butter leaf lettuce	3 cups	21	2 g	2 g
Cabbage (red or green)	1 cup, chopped	18	1 g	2 g
Carrots	1 cup, chopped	50	1 g	4 g
Cauliflower	1 cup	25	2 g	2.5 g
Celery	2 sticks (7" each)	13	0.6 g	1.3 g
Corn	½ cup	89	3 g	2 g
Cucumber	½ cup, sliced	8	0.3 g	0.3 g
Eggplant	1 cup, sliced with peel	20	1 g	3 g
Grape tomatoes	1 cup	25	2 g	2 g
Kale	1 cup, chopped	34	2 g	1.3 g
Lima beans	½ cup	105	6 g	5 g
Mixed baby greens	3 cups	22	2 g	2 g
Mushrooms	1 cup, sliced	21	3 g	1 g
Onion	¼ cup, chopped	16	0.4 g	0.7 g
Peas	½ cup	62	4 g	4 g
Radishes	½ cup, sliced	9	0.7 g	1 g
Romaine lettuce	3 cups	29	2 g	4 g
Russet potato	1 medium with skin	188	5 g	3 g
Scallions	¼ cup, chopped	8	0.5 g	0.7 g
Shallots	¼ cup, chopped	29	1 g	0.7 g
Sweet potato	½ cup or ½ medium potato with skin	81	2 g	3 g
Tomatoes	1 cup, chopped	32	2 g	2 g
Tomatoes, canned stewed (no-salt-added)	¼ cup	40	2 g	1 g

Fruits

FOOD	SERVING SIZE	CALORIES	PROTEIN	FIBER
Apple	1 medium	72	0.4 g	3 g
Banana	1 medium	105	1.3 g	3 g
Blackberries	1 cup	62	2 g	8 g
Blueberries	1 cup	83	1 g	3.5 g
Cantaloupe	1 cup, cubed	54	1.3 g	1.4 g
Clementine or tangerine	1 medium	47	0.7 g	1.6 g
Cranberries, dried	2 Tbsp	47	0 g	1 g
Currants	2 Tbsp	25	0.4 g	0.6 g
Figs, dried	2 (about 2 Tbsp)	46	0.6 g	2 g
Honeydew	1 cup, cubed	64	1 g	1.4 g
Peach or nectarine	1 medium	59	1.4 g	2.3 g
Pear	1 medium	96	0.6 g	5 g
Pineapple	½ cup canned, chopped	39	0.5 g	1 g
Raisins	2 Tbsp	54	0.6 g	0.7 g
Raspberries	1 cup	64	1.5 g	8 g
Strawberries	1 cup	46	1 g	3 g

Grains

FOOD	SERVING SIZE	CALORIES	PROTEIN	FIBER
Baked potato chips	1 oz	133	0.7 g	1 g
Bread, whole wheat	1-oz slice	80	4 g	2 g
Brown rice, cooked	½ cup	109	2 g	1.8 g
Cream of Wheat cereal* (instant), dry	¼ cup	160	5 g	1.6 g
English muffin, whole wheat	1 (2 oz)	134	6 g	4 g
Kashi Good Friends cereal*	¼ cup	43	1 g	3 g
Oatmeal (quick or old-fashioned), dry	¼ cup	152	7 g	4 g
Pasta, whole wheat (any shape), cooked	½ cup	87	4 g	2 g
Pita, whole wheat	1 pita (6")	111	5 g	4 g
Quinoa, cooked	½ cup	111	4 g	2.6 g
Rice, wild, cooked	½ cup	83	3 g	1.5 g

FOOD	SERVING SIZE	CALORIES	PROTEIN	FIBER
Tortilla, soft, whole grain	1 tortilla (8")	140	9 g	6 g
Tortilla chips, baked	1 oz	110	3 g	2 g
Vegetable chips, baked	1 oz	160	1 g	3 g
Waffle, whole grain	1	90	2 g	1.5 g
Wasa multigrain cracker*	1	45	2 g	2 g

The nutrition values for these foods will vary according to brand. Please use these values as a goal when selecting your product.

Step 3: Account for Any Added Ingredients

Even small amounts of dressings, flavorings, or other fixings added to your main ingredients can contribute to higher-than-realized calorie counts. Consistently underestimating your calorie intake by even 20 percent (that's just 80 calories in a 400-calorie meal, or the equivalent of 2 teaspoons of olive oil) can keep you from losing 20 pounds over the course of a year.

Healthy Fats

FOOD	SERVING SIZE	CALORIES	PROTEIN	FIBER
Almond butter	1 Tbsp	101	2.4 g	0.6 g
Almonds	1 Tbsp, slivered	39	1.4 g	0.8 g
Avocado	¼ cup, chopped	58	1.1 g	4 g
Canola oil	1 tsp	40	0 g	0 g
Cashews	1 Tbsp	49	1.3 g	0.3 g
Olive oil	1 tsp	40	0 g	0 g
Olives (black or green)	5 large	25	0.2 g	0.7 g
Peanut butter	1 Tbsp	94	4 g	1 g
Peanuts	1 Tbsp	52	2.4 g	0.7 g
Pecans	1 Tbsp	47	0.6 g	0.7 g
Pine nuts	1 Tbsp	58	1.2 g	0.3 g
Pistachios	1 Tbsp	44	2 g	0.8 g
Sesame oil	1 tsp	40	0 g	0 g
Walnuts	1 Tbsp, chopped	48	2 g	0.5 g

Condiments and Sweeteners

FOOD	SERVING SIZE	CALORIES	PROTEIN	FIBER
All-fruit jam or jelly	1 Tbsp	35	0 g	Up to 3 g
Bread crumbs (plain)	2 Tbsp	53	2 g	0.6 g
Brown sugar, granulated	1 tsp	11	0 g	0 g
Capers	1 tsp	0.7	0 g	0 g
Chocolate chips, semisweet or dark	1 Tbsp	52	0.5 g	0.6 g
Chocolate syrup	1 Tbsp	52	0.4 g	0 g
Confectioners' sugar	1 tsp	10	0 g	0 g
Honey	1 tsp	21	0 g	0 g
Light mayonnaise	1 Tbsp	49	0 g	0 g
Low-sodium vegetable or chicken broth	½ cup	10	1.2 g	0.5 g
Maple syrup	1 Tbsp	52	0 g	0 g
Parmesan cheese	1 Tbsp	22	2 g	0 g
Reduced-fat cream cheese	2 Tbsp	70	2 g	0 g
Reduced-fat feta cheese	1 oz	50	6 g	0 g
Reduced-fat sour cream	2 Tbsp	45	1 g	0 g
Salsa	2 Tbsp	9	0.5 g	0.5 g
Spaghetti sauce	½ cup	61	1.5 g	2 g
White sugar, granulated	1 tsp	16	0 g	0 g

Sample Meal Ideas

Here are some examples of how you can use the steps above to make a meal that suits this plan.

YOU WANT: YOGURT FOR BREAKFAST

Step 1: Start with 1¼ cups fat-free yogurt (171.25 calories, 17.5 g protein, 0 g fiber).

Step 2: Stir in 2 dried figs, chopped (46 calories, 0.6 g protein, 2 g fiber), and pair it with 3 Wasa multigrain crackers (135 calories, 6 g protein, 6 g fiber).

Step 3: Top it off with a tablespoon of pecans (47 calories, 0.6 g protein, 0.7 g fiber).

Step 4: Check your total nutrition goals: **399.25 calories, 24.7 g protein, 8.7 g fiber**

YOU WANT: A SANDWICH FOR LUNCH

Step 1: Start with a Boca Burger (100 calories, 19 g protein, 6 g fiber).

Step 2: Choose a bun for your burger, such as a whole wheat pita (111 calories, 5 g protein, 4 g fiber).

Step 3: You have calories to spare, so add a side of 1 ounce baked tortilla chips (110 calories, 3 g protein, 2 g fiber), topped with 2 tablespoons of salsa (9 calories, 0.5 g protein, 0.5 g fiber). Have an apple (72 calories, 0.4 g protein, 3 g fiber).

Step 4: Check your total nutrition goals: **402 calories, 27.9 g protein, 15.5 g fiber**

Did You Know? Herbs and Spices

Dried and fresh herbs and spices can be rich in antioxidants and are a great addition to any meal. Herbs are very low in calories, as are extracts such as vanilla and condiments such as lemon or lime juice, mustard, vinegar, garlic, and cooking spray. Feel free to incorporate as needed.

YOU WANT: FISH FOR DINNER

Step 1: Start with 3 ounces broiled salmon (120 calories, 17 g protein, 0 g fiber)

Step 2: Serve it with a side of ½ cup cooked corn (89 calories, 3 g protein, 2 g fiber) and ½ cup cooked peas (62 calories, 4 g protein, 4 g fiber). Have 1 cup strawberries for dessert (46 calories, 1 g protein, 3 g fiber).

Step 3: Account for 2 teaspoons olive oil used in cooking (herbs and vinegar are freebies) (80 calories, 0 g protein, 0 g fiber).

Step 4: Check your total nutrition goals: **397 calories, 25 g protein, 9 g fiber**

○ **Helpful Hints:** Guidelines for Canned Foods

Canned foods such as beans, fish, tomatoes, and soups can be very healthy options. But they can also pack a surprising amount of sodium. With any canned foods you buy, scan the labels to choose the lowest-sodium option available, opting for no-salt-added foods whenever possible. You can also rinse and drain solid foods (from tuna to sweet corn) canned in a bit of liquid. If you do select a no-salt-added food, you may want to remove the storage liquid, particularly with canned beans, which can be a bit "gunky." It may seem obvious, but don't attempt to rinse soups, which are mostly liquid, because you'll rinse away the whole product!

If you can't find no-salt-added canned solid foods, look for the one with the least sodium you can find, and follow these instructions to remove about 30 percent of the sodium.

○ Place food in a colander in the sink.

○ Rinse under cool, running water for at least 3 minutes.

○ Allow the food to drain for 1 to 2 minutes.

Rinsing your food for longer does not remove more sodium than this, so there's no need to rinse for more than 3 minutes.

Keep in mind that you may not want to rinse some canned foods, such as tomatoes, because the liquid contributes to the recipe, so always follow your recipe instructions for this.

YOU WANT: A SAVORY SNACK

Step 1: Start with 3 ounces chunk light tuna packed in water (90 calories, 20 g protein, 0 g fiber).

Step 2: Add ½ cup cooked whole wheat pasta for fiber (87 calories, 4 g protein, 2 g fiber).

Step 3: Toss with ½ teaspoon olive oil (20 calories, 0 g protein, 0 g fiber), a splash of white vinegar (freebie), and 1 teaspoon dried parsley (freebie).

Step 4: Check your total nutrition goals: **197 calories, 24 g protein, 2 g fiber**

YOU WANT: A FRUIT SMOOTHIE

Step 1: Choose a protein base, like a cup of fat-free soy milk (70 calories, 6 g protein, 0.5 g fiber) and ½ cup 0% Greek yogurt (50 calories, 8 g protein, 0 g fiber).

Step 2: Add a cup of blackberries (62 calories, 2 g protein, 8 g fiber).

Step 3: Add ½ teaspoon vanilla extract (a freebie).

Step 4: Check your total nutrition goals: **182 calories, 16 g protein, 8.5 g fiber**

YOU WANT: A CHOCOLATY SNACK

Step 1: Start with 1 cup 0% Greek yogurt (100 calories, 16 g protein, 0 g fiber).

Step 2: Add some fruit for fiber, such as 1 cup strawberries (46 calories, 1 g protein, 3 g fiber).

Step 3: Add 1 tablespoon chocolate chips (52 calories, 0.5 g protein, 0.6 g fiber).

Step 4: Check your total nutrition goals: **198 calories, 17.5 g protein, 3.6 g fiber**

Tone Every Inch Recipes

The recipes that follow meet all of the nutrition goals for this program—no math required. They offer a mix of meals for one as well as meals that you can share with friends or family (or save for leftovers). All of the meals include about 400 calories and are packed with at least 20 grams of protein and 8 grams of fiber, so they are all interchangeable (that's right, if you want to have breakfast for dinner, we won't say anything!). The snacks are each about 200 calories and include 15 grams of protein and 2 grams of fiber.

Breakfast

If you're planning to do your workout first thing in the morning, look for a recipe with a "Breakaway Breakfast Option." To ensure you have enough energy to give it your all, eat whatever is described before you go out for your workout. Then finish up your breakfast when you're done.

Hot Cereal with Cashews and Berries

Makes 4 servings

Prep Time: 5 minutes | Total Time: 15 minutes

1 pound silken tofu

4 cups fat-free milk

¾ cup uncooked whole wheat farina (such as Cream of Wheat)

3 tablespoons chopped cashews

1½ tablespoons honey

5 cups fresh or frozen and thawed unsweetened mixed berries

1. Place the tofu in a blender and pulse just until pureed. Set aside.

2. In a saucepan, bring the milk to a boil over medium heat. Stir in the farina and whisk until smooth.

3. Reduce the heat to low. Add the tofu and cook, stirring, for 2½ minutes.

4. Remove from the heat. Stir in the cashews and honey. Top with the berries.

Breakaway Breakfast Option: Have the berries from your serving of cereal (1¼ cups) plus 2 teaspoons cashews.

....

Per serving: 382 calories, 20 g protein, 64 g carbohydrates, 6 g total fat, 1 g saturated fat, 8 g fiber, 106 mg sodium

Did You Know? The Power of a Protein-Packed Breakfast

You probably know that breakfast is good for you. But plenty of women skip it anyway, whether because of busy schedules or a (misguided) attempt to cut calories by eliminating meals. (Unfortunately, research shows that skipping meals will lead you to eat all of those missing calories and more when you get hungry later.) It turns out that getting a dose of protein first thing in the morning is the best way to keep cravings in check throughout the day, according to a study by researchers at the University of Missouri at Columbia.

When habitual breakfast skippers ate one of two breakfasts with an identical number of calories—either an ordinary bowl of cereal with milk or a high-protein waffle and yogurt combo—the ones who fueled with protein felt less famished before lunch. After eating their designated breakfasts for a week, the subjects filled out questionnaires rating their hunger and satiety. Then they underwent MRI scans of their brains. Not only did the high-protein diners feel fuller over the course of the week, but when scientists took a peek at their brain activity, they saw less activity in the areas of the brain related to reward-seeking behavior (read: the part of your brain that's likely to make you reach for a Snickers instead of an apple).

Cinnamon Pecan Oatmeal

Makes 4 servings

Prep Time: 5 minutes | Total Time: 20 minutes

3 tablespoons chopped pecans

3¾ cups water

2 cups quick-cooking oats

4 apples, thinly sliced, divided

1 teaspoon cinnamon

2 teaspoons vanilla extract

2 teaspoons honey

4 cups 0% plain Greek yogurt

1. Preheat the oven to 350°F. Spread the pecans on a baking sheet and toast for 4 minutes, or until browned.

2. In a large saucepan, heat the water until boiling. Add the oats and 1 apple. Reduce the heat to low and simmer, stirring occasionally, for 3 minutes, or until thickened.

3. Remove from the heat and stir in the cinnamon, vanilla, honey, and pecans. Top with the remaining apples.

4. Serve each portion with 1 cup yogurt.

Speed-it-up tip: For an early morning meal, nuts can be toasted the night before. Store them at room temperature in a resealable plastic bag for a few days, but if you're toasting a big batch, it's best to store them sealed in a bag in the freezer.

Breakaway Breakfast Option: Have 1 apple and 1 cup 0% plain Greek yogurt.

Per serving: 432 calories, 27 g protein, 67 g carbohydrates, 7 g total fat, 0.5 g saturated fat, 10 g fiber, 87 mg sodium

➲ **Helpful Hints:** Speed Up Your Slow-Cooked Oats

If you're like me and think slow-cooked oatmeal beats the instant kind hands-down (and that steel-cut is better still), try this fast method for slow-cooked taste. The night before, boil 4 cups of water in a pot and add 1 cup of steel-cut oatmeal (double the measurements if you want more leftovers). Simmer the mixture for 1 minute, and then cover the pot and store it overnight in the refrigerator. The next morning, heat the oatmeal on low heat for 9 to 12 minutes, stirring occasionally. Serve the oatmeal you want to have now, and allow the remainder to cool. Leftovers can be stored in the refrigerator for up to 5 days, or frozen in easy-to-reheat individual portions for up to 3 months.

Spinach and Feta Omelet

Makes 2 servings

Prep Time: 10 minutes | Total Time: 30 minutes

2 eggs

½ cup egg whites

¼ cup fat-free milk

½ teaspoon dried basil

1½ teaspoons olive oil

1½ cups spinach leaves

1 scallion, green and white parts, thinly sliced

1 ounce reduced-fat feta cheese

1 pear, thinly sliced

4 slices whole wheat bread, toasted

2 teaspoons all-fruit jam

1. In a large bowl, whisk together the eggs, egg whites, milk, and basil. Heat the oil in a large skillet and pour in the egg mixture. Stir constantly with a heatproof rubber spatula for 15 seconds, or until the eggs thicken to a custardy consistency.

2. Tilt the pan to allow any uncooked eggs to run to the side. Run the spatula all around the edge of the omelet.

3. Top with the spinach, scallions, and feta. Fold the other half of the omelet over the cheese. Turn off the heat and let stand for 30 seconds to set around filling. Cut into half. With the spatula, gently push one-half of the omelet onto each of 2 plates.

4. Serve each omelet with half of the pear slices and 2 slices whole wheat toast, each spread with ½ teaspoon jam.

Breakaway Breakfast Option: Have one-half thinly sliced pear and 1 slice whole wheat toast spread with ½ teaspoon all-fruit jam.

Per serving: 378 calories, 23 g protein, 47 g carbohydrates, 12 g total fat, 4 g saturated fat, 8 g fiber, 623 mg sodium

Fried Egg Wrap

Makes 4 servings

Prep Time: 10 minutes | Total Time: 25 minutes

2 tablespoons olive oil, divided

4 eggs

4 tablespoons chopped onion

4 whole wheat wraps (about 120 calories each with at least 6 grams fiber)

2 medium tomatoes, sliced

Black pepper

4 cups 0% plain Greek yogurt

4 cups fresh or frozen and thawed unsweetened strawberries

1. Heat 1 tablespoon of the oil in a skillet over medium heat. Crack 2 eggs into the skillet. Cook for 3 minutes, or until set. Remove to a plate.

2. Add the remaining 1 tablespoon oil to the skillet and repeat with the remaining 2 eggs. Remove to the plate.

3. Coat the same skillet with cooking spray. Cook the onion, stirring frequently, for 5 minutes, or until translucent.

4. Fill each wrap with 1 egg and one-quarter of the tomatoes and onion. Sprinkle with black pepper to taste.

5. Serve each portion with 1 cup Greek yogurt and 1 cup strawberries.

Breakaway Breakfast Option: Have ½ cup 0% Greek yogurt and ½ cup strawberries.

....

Per serving: 406 calories, 40 g protein, 42 g carbohydrates, 16 g total fat, 2.5 g saturated fat, 16 g fiber, 482 mg sodium

Blackberry Nut Smoothie

Makes 1 servings

Prep Time: 5 minutes | Total Time: 5 minutes

2 cups fat-free milk

1 cup frozen unsweetened blackberries

1 tablespoon almond or peanut butter

2 teaspoons honey

Place the milk, blackberries, nut butter, and honey in a blender and blend until smooth. Serve immediately.

Breakaway Breakfast Option: Have 1 cup fat-free milk with 1/4 cup frozen and thawed unsweetened blackberries.

Per serving: 402 calories, 21 g protein, 62 g carbohydrates, 10 g total fat, 1 g saturated fat, 8 g fiber, 277 mg sodium

 Helpful Hints: Speed Up Your Smoothies

To save time in the morning and to avoid waking up the whole house with a blender, you can make most smoothies in advance. The night before, blend your smoothie and store it in a covered container in the refrigerator. If you don't have a tight-fitting lid, cover it with plastic wrap or foil. Smoothies that include just milk and fruit will be a bit more watery the next day. Smoothies with yogurt and fruit tend to be a little thicker and store nicely for a good consistency the next day. Either way, you'll want to shake or stir the ingredients before you sip.

Maple Cashew Smoothie

Makes 1 servings

Prep Time: 5 minutes | Total Time: 5 minutes plus overnight
soaking time for cashews

2 tablespoons raw cashews

1 small banana

2 teaspoons maple syrup

1 cup 0% plain Greek yogurt

1½ cups frozen unsweetened
strawberries

1. Soak the cashews in ½ cup of water in the refrigerator overnight (they'll be easier to blend).

2. Drain the cashews, discarding the liquid. Place the cashews, banana, syrup, yogurt, and strawberries in a blender and blend until smooth. Serve immediately.

Breakaway Breakfast Option: Have 1/2 cup 0% Greek yogurt with 1/2 cup frozen and thawed unsweetened strawberries.

Per serving: 415 calories, 29 g protein, 66 g carbohydrates, 7 g total fat, 1 g saturated fat, 8 g fiber, 115 mg sodium

Apple and Pear Melt

Makes 4 servings

Prep Time: 5 minutes | Total Time: 10 minutes

2 cups fat-free ricotta cheese

2 tablespoons honey

1 teaspoon vanilla extract

4 whole wheat pitas (6″ diameter)

1½ cups sliced pears

1½ cups sliced apples

6 tablespoons pecans

1. Preheat the oven to 375°F. Coat a baking sheet with cooking spray.

2. In a medium bowl, combine the ricotta, honey, and vanilla. Spread one-quarter of the mixture into each pita. Stuff with one-quarter of the pears, apples, and pecans. Place on the baking sheet.

3. Bake for 6 minutes, or until heated through.

Breakaway Breakfast Option: Have one-half of the pita as an open-faced sandwich.

Per serving: 411 calories, 23 g protein, 65 g carbohydrates, 8 g total fat, 1 g saturated fat, 8 g fiber, 502 mg sodium

Quinoa "Quiche"

Makes 4 servings

Prep Time: 10 minutes | Total Time: 45 minutes

4 cups water

1¼ cups quinoa, rinsed well

1½ pounds silken tofu

2 tablespoons chopped shallot

2 tablespoons canola oil

4 cups spinach

3 tablespoons fresh rosemary, chopped

½ teaspoon salt

1⅓ cups raspberries

1 cup fat-free plain yogurt

1. Preheat the oven to 350°F. Coat a 12" pie plate with cooking spray. Bring the water to a boil. Add the quinoa and boil for 5 minutes. Drain and remove quinoa to a large bowl.

2. In a food processor, combine the tofu, shallot, and oil. Process for 2 minutes, or until smooth.

3. Add to the quinoa and stir in the spinach, rosemary, and salt. Stir just until blended. Pour into the pan. Bake for 30 minutes, or until set.

4. Serve each portion with ⅓ cup raspberries topped with ¼ cup yogurt.

....

Per serving: 425 calories, 20 g protein, 52 g carbohydrates, 16 g total fat, 1 g saturated fat, 18 g fiber, 377 mg sodium

Raisin Bran Muffins

Makes 12 muffins

Prep Time: 15 minutes | Total Time: 29 minutes

1 cup bran flake cereal, lightly crushed

1 cup rolled oats

1 cup whole wheat flour

2 tablespoons brown sugar

2 tablespoons granulated sugar

¼ cup ground flaxseed

1 tablespoon baking powder

1 teaspoon ground nutmeg

1 teaspoon ground cinnamon

¼ teaspoon salt

1 cup fat-free milk

½ cup egg whites (about 6 egg whites)

¼ cup honey

3 tablespoons canola oil

¾ cup golden or dark raisins

4 cups fat-free ricotta cheese

1 cup peanut butter

4 cups fresh or frozen and thawed unsweetened raspberries

1. Preheat the oven to 400°F. Coat a 12-cup muffin tin with cooking spray or use muffin liners.

2. In a large bowl, combine the cereal, oats, flour, sugars, flaxseed, baking powder, nutmeg, cinnamon, and salt. Add the milk, egg whites, honey, and oil. Stir until just moistened. Fold in the raisins.

3. Evenly divide the batter among the muffin cups. Bake for 12 to 14 minutes, or until a wooden pick inserted in the center comes out clean.

4. Mix together the ricotta cheese and peanut butter.

5. Serve each muffin spread with about ⅓ cup of the ricotta cheese mixture plus ⅓ cup raspberries on the side.

....

Per muffin: 424 calories, 25 g protein, 51 g carbohydrates, 16 g total fat, 3 g saturated fat, 8 g fiber, 408 mg sodium

Eggplant Pizzas

Makes 4 servings

Prep Time: 10 minutes | Total Time: 25 minutes

4 whole wheat English muffins, halved

4 eggs

¼ cup dried bread crumbs

½ eggplant, sliced

1 tablespoon olive oil

¾ cup low-sodium spaghetti sauce

1 cup shredded reduced-fat mozzarella cheese

1. Preheat the oven to 350°F. Coat a baking sheet with cooking spray. Place the muffins on the sheet.

2. In a shallow bowl, lightly beat the eggs. Place the bread crumbs in another shallow bowl. Dip the eggplant slices in the egg, then coat in the bread crumbs.

3. Heat the oil in a skillet over medium heat. Cook the eggplant slices for 5 minutes, turning once, or until golden brown.

4. Divide the sauce, eggplant slices, and cheese among the muffins. Bake for 10 minutes, or until the cheese melts and the muffins are toasted.

Breakaway Breakfast Option: Have one of your pizzas (one English muffin half).

Per serving: 388 calories, 23 g protein, 43 g carbohydrates, 16 g total fat, 5 g saturated fat, 8 g fiber, 652 mg sodium

Lunch and Dinner

Whether you brown-bag your lunch (or your dinner) or cook it fresh, the options that follow will fulfill your nutritional needs at noon or in the evening. As you plan your day, remember that eating either a meal or a snack within an hour of your workout will help to make sure your muscles have the protein they need to get strong and sculpted.

Savory Tuna Sandwich

Makes 4 servings

Prep Time: 10 minutes | Total Time: 10 minutes

16 ounces low-sodium chunk light tuna, drained

6 medium black olives, chopped

2 teaspoons capers, drained

¼ cup white vinegar

1 tablespoon olive oil

8 slices whole wheat bread

2 cups arugula

4 large oranges

1. In a medium bowl, toss together the tuna, olives, capers, vinegar, and oil.

2. Spread the tuna mixture on 4 slices of the bread and top each with ½ cup arugula. Top with the remaining bread slices.

3. Serve each sandwich with 1 large orange.

Per serving: 385 calories, 39 g protein, 40 g carbohydrates, 8 g total fat, 1 g saturated fat, 8 g fiber, 438 mg sodium

Portobello Sandwich

Makes 4 servings

Prep Time: 10 minutes | Total Time: 25 minutes

4 teaspoons canola oil, divided

1 shallot, minced

4 portobello mushroom caps

1 cup 2% shredded mozzarella cheese

1 cup 0% plain Greek yogurt, divided

1 tablespoon chopped fresh parsley

4 whole wheat rolls (about 160 calories each), split

2 cups mixed baby greens

2 teaspoons maple syrup

8 crispbread-style whole wheat crackers

1. Heat 1 teaspoon of the oil in a nonstick skillet over medium heat. Add the shallot and cook, stirring frequently, for 2 minutes. Transfer to a small bowl.

2. Add the remaining 3 teaspoons oil to the skillet and cook the mushrooms for 5 minutes, turning once, or until tender. Turn off the heat and top each mushroom with ¼ cup mozzarella; allow the cheese to melt.

3. Mix the shallot with ½ cup of the yogurt and the parsley.

4. Spread the bottom of each roll with 2 tablespoons of the yogurt mixture. Top with 1 mushroom and ½ cup greens. Top with the top halves of the rolls.

5. In a small bowl, combine the remaining ½ cup yogurt and the syrup. Serve each sandwich with 2 crackers each spread with 1 tablespoon of the yogurt mixture.

Per serving: 425 calories, 21 g protein, 57 g carbohydrates, 15 g total fat, 5 g saturated fat, 8 g fiber, 594 mg sodium

Zuppa Italiano

Makes 4 servings

Prep Time: 10 minutes | Total Time: 30 minutes

2 teaspoons olive oil

¾ pound 95% lean ground beef

5 cups low-sodium beef broth

½ teaspoon dried basil

½ teaspoon dried oregano

½ teaspoon dried rosemary

¼ teaspoon onion powder

⅛ teaspoon garlic powder

1 cup whole wheat macaroni or other small pasta

1 can (16 ounces) no-salt-added stewed tomatoes

1 can (15.5 ounces) no-salt-added kidney beans, rinsed and drained

1. In a large saucepan, heat the oil over medium heat and cook the ground beef for 5 minutes, stirring, or until browned.

2. Stir in the broth, basil, oregano, rosemary, onion powder, and garlic powder. Cover and bring to a boil.

3. Stir in the pasta and return to a boil. Reduce the heat to low, cover, and simmer for 8 minutes, or until the pasta is tender.

4. Stir in the tomatoes and beans and return to a boil. Cook for 1 minute, or until heated through.

....

Per serving: 399 calories, 39 g protein, 38 g carbohydrates, 10 g total fat, 3.5 g saturated fat, 10 g fiber, 164 mg sodium

Vegetable Chicken Chowder

Makes 4 servings

Prep Time: 15 minutes | Total Time: 45 minutes

4 cups low-sodium chicken broth

2 cups baby carrots, chopped (about 30)

1 cup chopped leeks

1 onion, chopped

¾ cup sliced mushrooms

¼ cup chopped shallots

2 teaspoons chopped fresh rosemary

1 clove garlic, minced

14 ounces boneless, skinless chicken breast, cut into ½" strips

3 tablespoons olive oil

3 tablespoons all-purpose flour

1 cup fat-free milk

2 cups fresh or frozen peas

1 tablespoon chopped fresh parsley

¼ teaspoon black pepper

1. Combine the broth, carrots, leeks, onion, mushrooms, shallots, rosemary, and garlic in a large saucepan. Bring to a boil. Reduce the heat to low, cover, and simmer for 20 minutes.

2. Remove half of the vegetables using a slotted spoon. Place in a blender or food processor and puree until smooth. Return to the saucepan.

3. Add the chicken and cook on low, covered, for 15 minutes, or until the chicken is no longer pink.

4. Meanwhile, heat the oil in a small saucepan over medium heat, stir in the flour until smooth, and cook for 2 minutes. Whisk in the milk, whisking constantly for 3 minutes, or until thickened.

5. Stir into the chicken mixture. Add the peas, parsley, and pepper. Cook for 5 minutes, or until the chowder is heated through and the peas are tender.

....

Per serving: 419 calories, 35 g protein, 38 g carbohydrates, 15 g total fat, 3 g saturated fat, 8 g fiber, 313 mg sodium

Spinach Salad with Tart Apple and Pecans

Makes 4 servings

Prep Time: 10 minutes | Total Time: 20 minutes

¼ cup red wine vinegar

2 tablespoons olive oil

⅛ teaspoon black pepper

10 cups baby spinach

4 medium Granny Smith apples, thinly sliced

¼ cup pecans

2 tablespoons chopped red onion

12 hard-boiled eggs, quartered (discard 4 yolks)

4 multigrain flatbread-style crackers

1. In a large bowl, whisk together the vinegar, oil, and pepper. Add the spinach, apples, pecans, and onion; toss to coat well. Divide into 4 salad bowls. Top each with 2 eggs and 1 egg white.

2. Serve each salad with 1 cracker.

....

Per serving: 444 calories, 21 g protein, 44 g carbohydrates, 22 g total fat, 8 g saturated fat, 10 g fiber, 358 mg sodium

Marinated Flank Steak and Chickpea Salad

Makes 4 servings

Prep Time: 5 minutes | Total Time: 20 minutes

3 tablespoons sherry vinegar

1½ tablespoons olive oil

1 tablespoon chopped fresh tarragon

⅛ teaspoon black pepper

1 can (15.5 ounces) chickpeas, rinsed and drained

2 cups grape tomatoes, halved

¾ pound flank steak, pierced with a fork several times and sliced into ¼"-thick slices

¼ cup chopped shallots

6 cups butter lettuce

1. In a large bowl, whisk together the vinegar, oil, tarragon, and pepper. Remove 1½ tablespoons of the vinaigrette and place in a medium bowl. Add the chickpeas and tomatoes to the medium bowl and stir to combine. Set aside.

2. Place the steak in the large bowl with the vinaigrette. Marinate for 10 minutes.

3. Coat a skillet with cooking spray and heat over medium-high heat. Cook the shallots, stirring, for 3 minutes, or until lightly browned. Add the steak and cook for 3 minutes, turning frequently.

4. Place 1½ cups of the lettuce on each of 4 plates. Top each with one-quarter of the chickpeas and tomatoes and one-quarter of the steak.

Per serving: 311 calories, 24 g protein, 24 g carbohydrates, 13 g total fat, 4 g saturated fat, 5 g fiber, 329 mg sodium

Teriyaki Chicken

Makes 4 servings

Prep Time: 10 minutes | Total Time: 45 minutes

1⅔ cups brown rice

2 teaspoons sesame oil

2 cups chopped onions

1½ cups fresh or frozen sliced carrots

1 cup fresh or frozen sliced mushrooms

½ pound boneless, skinless chicken breast, sliced into strips

½ cup sliced scallions

2 tablespoons low-sodium teriyaki sauce

2 teaspoons minced garlic

1. Prepare the rice according to package directions.

2. Meanwhile, heat the oil in a skillet over medium heat. Cook the onions, carrots, and mushrooms, stirring frequently, for 5 minutes.

3. Add the chicken, scallions, teriyaki sauce, and garlic to the pan. Cook for 5 minutes, stirring often, or until chicken is no longer pink.

4. Divide the rice among 4 plates. Divide the vegetable-chicken mixture over the rice.

....

Per serving: 423 calories, 20 g protein, 72 g carbohydrates, 6 g total fat, 1 g saturated fat, 8 g fiber, 236 mg sodium

 Helpful Hints: Speed Up Weeknight Meals

Cooking rice (especially the long-grain variety) can be time consuming. To save time on busy days, you can make it in advance and store portions in the freezer. When you're ready to use it, add a splash of water—about 2 teaspoons' worth per 2 cups of cooked rice—and reheat it in the microwave. (Be sure to use a lid so the rice doesn't dry out.) Cook for 1 minute on high per 2 cups of rice, stir, and repeat if necessary. When heated in an airtight container with a little water, the rice is steamed a bit, allowing the dry pieces of rice to absorb moisture and fluff up.

➲ Helpful Hints: DIY Bread Crumbs

Of course, you can buy a can of bread crumbs at the store, but making your own is an easy way to use up the end of a leftover loaf. Preheat the oven to 200°F. Coat a baking sheet with cooking spray. Remove the crusts from each slice of bread and place the slices on the baking sheet, being careful not to overlap them. Bake for 30 minutes and then allow to cool. Break the bread into smaller pieces. Put the pieces in a food processor and blend for 30 seconds. Spread the crumbs over the baking sheet and bake for 5 minutes. Allow to cool. Store the crumbs in an airtight container or resealable plastic bag (don't forget to label it with the date) in the freezer for up to 2 months. Four slices of bread will make about 1 cup of dried bread crumbs.

Roasted Penne with Fish and Cabbage

Makes 4 servings

Prep Time: 10 minutes | Total Time: 50 minutes

8 ounces whole wheat penne (about 2¼ cups)

1 tablespoon olive oil

5 cups thinly sliced cabbage

1 red onion, chopped

½ teaspoon caraway seeds

6 ounces mackerel

1 cup chopped scallions

¼ cup dry bread crumbs

2 tablespoons Dijon mustard

1. Prepare the pasta according to package directions.

2. Meanwhile, preheat the oven to 400°F. Coat a 13" x 9" baking dish with cooking spray.

3. Heat the oil in a large skillet over medium heat. Add the cabbage, onion, and caraway seeds and cook for 5 minutes, stirring occasionally, or until lightly browned. Cover the pan, reduce the heat to low, and cook for 5 minutes, or until tender. Stir in the pasta and toss to combine.

4. Pour the mixture into the baking dish and top with the mackerel.

5. In a bowl, combine the scallions, bread crumbs, and mustard. Spread the mixture evenly over the top of the mackerel and pasta.

6. Bake for 20 minutes.

Per serving: 394 calories, 20 g protein, 50 g carbohydrates, 13 g total fat, 2.5 g saturated fat, 12 g fiber, 221 mg sodium

Turkey and Sprouts with Dill Spread

Makes 4 servings

Prep Time: 10 minutes | Total Time: 10 minutes

4 whole wheat high-fiber tortillas

4 tablespoons reduced-fat cream cheese

1 teaspoon dried dill

½ pound reduced-sodium turkey breast

2 cups alfalfa sprouts

2 medium apples, thinly sliced

4 ounces baked vegetable chips

1. Spread each tortilla with 1 tablespoon of the cream cheese and sprinkle with ¼ teaspoon of the dill.

2. Top each tortilla with 2 ounces of turkey breast, ½ cup of sprouts, and half an apple. Roll up to eat.

3. Serve each tortilla with 1 ounce of chips.

Per serving: 370 calories, 24 g protein, 45 g carbohydrates, 13 g total fat, 2 g saturated fat, 12 g fiber, 927 mg sodium

⟳ Helpful Hints: Save the Sauce!

If you have leftover pesto or broth, don't toss it, freeze it! Pour the remainder into an ice cube tray. Once frozen solid, after about 2 hours, pop the cubes into a resealable plastic bag and place back in the freezer. Don't forget to put the date on the bag, and use within 3 months for the very best taste. These small portions are just right for topping a meal later, such as a side of pasta or rice or even a piece of chicken breast. To defrost, use the defrost setting on your microwave for 30 to 45 seconds per ice cube–size portion, or just toss it into the cooking pan.

Basil Pesto Salmon

Makes 4 servings

Prep Time: 20 minutes | Total Time: 50 minutes

1 cup wild rice

1½ cups fresh basil leaves

¼ cup low-sodium chicken broth

1 tablespoon slivered almonds

1 tablespoon pine nuts

1 tablespoon lemon juice

1 tablespoon grated Parmesan cheese

1 tablespoon + 2 teaspoons olive oil, divided

2 teaspoons minced garlic

¼ teaspoon black pepper

1 pound salmon

2½ cups raspberries

½ cup chopped parsley

1. Cook the rice according to package directions.

2. Meanwhile, preheat the oven to 350°F. Coat a baking sheet with cooking spray.

3. In a food processor, combine the basil, broth, almonds, pine nuts, lemon juice, cheese, 1 tablespoon of the oil, garlic, and pepper. Process until smooth.

4. Spoon 3 tablespoons of the pesto mixture over 1 side of the salmon, and 3 tablespoons of pesto on the other side. Place the salmon on the baking sheet. Bake for 10 minutes, or until just opaque.

5. Toss the rice with the remaining 2 teaspoons of oil, raspberries, and parsley. Serve the salmon with the rice on the side.

Per serving: 416 calories, 30 g protein, 38 g carbohydrates, 17 g total fat, 2.5 g saturated fat, 8 g fiber, 83 mg sodium

Pork Tenderloin
with Red Pear Relish

Makes 4 servings

Prep Time: 25 minutes | Total Time: 45 minutes

1 cup brown rice

2 teaspoons canola oil

1 red onion, sliced

4 red pears, cored and sliced

1 tablespoon sherry vinegar

1 teaspoon chopped fresh sage

¼ teaspoon salt

¾ pound pork tenderloin, sliced into ¾"-thick slices

1. Cook the rice according to package directions and set aside.

2. Twenty minutes before the rice is finished, heat the oil in a large skillet over medium heat. Cook the onion for 5 minutes. Add the pears, vinegar, sage, and salt and cook for 10 minutes, stirring often. Remove mixture to a bowl.

3. Coat the pan with cooking spray and add the pork. Cook for 8 minutes, turning once, or until no longer pink.

4. Divide the rice among 4 plates. Divide the pork mixture over the rice.

Per serving: 395 calories, 22 g protein, 65 g carbohydrates, 6 g total fat, 1 g saturated fat, 9 g fiber, 216 mg sodium

Beef Tenderloin with Tomatoes and Spinach

Makes 4 servings

Prep Time: 20 minutes | Total Time: 20 minutes

2 teaspoons + 1 tablespoon olive oil, divided

6 cups baby spinach

4 large tomatoes, chopped

3 tablespoons balsamic vinegar

2 teaspoons minced garlic

¼ teaspoon salt

¼ teaspoon black pepper

¾ pound beef tenderloin, sliced into 4 slices

2 cans (15.5 ounces each) no-salt-added cannellini beans, rinsed and drained

1. Heat 2 teaspoons of the oil in a large skillet over medium heat. Add the spinach, tomatoes, vinegar, garlic, salt, and pepper. Cook, stirring constantly, for 3 minutes, or until the spinach is wilted. Remove to a bowl.

2. Heat the remaining 1 tablespoon of oil to the skillet. Add the steak and cook for 4 minutes, turning once. Place 1 steak slice on each of 4 plates.

3. Return the spinach mixture to the skillet and add the cannellini beans. Heat for 3 minutes, or until heated through. Serve alongside the steak.

Per serving: 414 calories, 27 g protein, 37 g carbohydrates, 18 g total fat, 5 g saturated fat, 11 g fiber, 306 mg sodium

Angel Hair and Vegetables

Makes 4 servings

Prep Time: 20 minutes | Total Time: 20 minutes

8 ounces whole wheat angel hair pasta (2¼ cups dry)

1½ tablespoons olive oil

¼ cup chopped shallots

2 teaspoons minced garlic

4 cups baby spinach

1 can (14.5 ounces) no-salt-added diced tomatoes1 cup sliced mushrooms

¼ teaspoon black pepper

⅛ teaspoon ground red pepper

1¼ cups reduced-fat feta cheese

1. Prepare the pasta according to package directions. Place in a large bowl.

2. Heat the oil in a large skillet over medium heat. Add the shallots and garlic and cook for 4 minutes.

3. Add the spinach, tomatoes, mushrooms, black pepper, and red pepper. Cook for 4 minutes, stirring constantly, or until the spinach begins to wilt.

4. Stir in the cheese and cook for 2 minutes, or until heated through. Pour over the pasta.

Per serving: 418 calories, 20 g protein, 56 g carbohydrates, 13 g total fat, 5 g saturated fat, 9 g fiber, 752 mg sodium

Lime Cilantro Black Beans

Makes 4 servings

Prep Time: 15 minutes | Total Time: 15 minutes

1½ cups chopped fresh cilantro

⅓ cup orange juice

1½ tablespoons lime juice

⅓ cup reduced-fat sour cream

½ teaspoon salt

3 cans (15.5 ounces each) no-salt-added canned black beans, rinsed and drained

⅓ cup chopped red onion

1 orange bell pepper, chopped

1 red bell pepper, chopped

1 avocado, diced

1. In a food processor, combine the cilantro, orange juice, lime juice, sour cream, and salt. Process until smooth.

2. In a large bowl, combine the beans, onion, peppers, and avocado. Toss with the cilantro mixture.

....

Per serving: 399 calories, 21 g protein, 58 g carbohydrates, 10 g total fat, 3 g saturated fat, 20 g fiber, 361 mg sodium

Tofu with Quinoa and Peas

Makes 4 servings

Prep Time: 10 minutes | Total Time: 40 minutes
plus time to drain tofu

1 tablespoon olive oil

1 pound firm tofu, drained and cut
into cubes

1 teaspoon paprika

1¾ cups low-sodium vegetable broth

1 cup + 1 tablespoon dry quinoa

1¼ cups spaghetti sauce

1 bag (10 ounces) frozen peas

1. Heat the oil in a skillet over medium heat. Add the tofu and cook for 7 minutes, tossing occasionally, or until brown on all sides.

2. Add the paprika and stir to coat the tofu. Stir in the broth and heat until boiling.

3. Stir in the quinoa. Reduce the heat to medium-low, cover, and cook for 15 minutes. Uncover, stir in the spaghetti sauce and peas, and cook for 5 minutes, stirring, or until the peas are heated through.

Per serving: 406 calories, 21 g protein, 50 g carbohydrates, 14 g total fat, 1 g saturated fat, 9 g fiber, 462 mg sodium

HOW TO DRAIN TOFU

If you're new to tofu, one simple technique can make all the difference: draining it. That's because tofu comes packed in liquid. It's perfect for using in smoothies this way, and you *can* cook with it as is, but the result will be a bit light and spongy—and a less-effective stand-in for meat. By taking a few minutes to drain it first, you'll get a meatier, chewier result in your finished dish. Once drained, the tofu can be stored in a covered container in your refrigerator for up to 7 days. Here's how to do it:

1. Put two paper towels in the bottom of a bowl, place the block of tofu on top, and cover with a cloth dish towel. The paper towels won't soak up all of the water, but they will help to absorb some of the water from the tofu.

2. Gently press on the dish towel to squeeze out some water.

3. The cloth dish towel will be wet; replace it with a fresh dish towel.

4. Balance a bowl or plate on top of the fresh dish towel to press down on the tofu. Keep this out of the way in your kitchen so you don't accidentally knock it over.

5. Let it sit for 15 minutes. Discard the paper towels and toss the dish towels in the laundry. Your tofu is now stir-fry ready!

White Bean Puttanesca

Makes 4 servings

Prep Time: 10 minutes | Total Time: 20 minutes

1 tablespoon olive oil

4 teaspoons minced garlic

4 anchovies canned in oil, drained and chopped

½ teaspoon dried rosemary

½ teaspoon dried oregano

1 can (14.5 ounces) no-salt-added diced tomatoes

1 tablespoon capers

1 cup low-salt spaghetti sauce

2 cans (15.5 ounces each) no-salt-added white beans, rinsed and drained

1. Heat the oil in a large skillet over medium heat. Add the garlic, anchovies, rosemary, and oregano and cook for 1 minute.

2. Reduce the heat to medium-low. Add the tomatoes, capers, spaghetti sauce, and beans and simmer for 10 minutes, stirring occasionally.

Per serving: 396 calories, 20 g protein, 66 g carbohydrates, 6 g total fat, 1.5 g saturated fat, 15 g fiber, 257 mg sodium

Snacks

Planning a satisfying bite for those times when hunger strikes can make all the difference between staying on track with your weight loss goals and heeding the siren call of the office vending machine. You can plan your snack for whatever time of day you need a pick-me-up, but if your usual workout time falls more than a couple of hours after your last meal, eating a snack first will help make sure you are fully fueled. Here are some options—sweet and savory—to keep cravings at bay.

Pistachio Fig Dip

Makes 4 servings

Prep Time: 5 minutes | Total Time: 5 minutes

1½ cups fat-free ricotta cheese

¼ cup pistachios

3 tablespoons chopped dried figs

8 flatbread-style whole wheat crackers (such as Wasa)

1. In a bowl, combine the ricotta, pistachios, and figs.

2. Divide into 4 portions and use as a dip with 2 crackers.

Per serving: 231 calories, 19 g protein, 34 g carbohydrates, 4 g total fat, 0.5 g saturated fat, 5 g fiber, 191 mg sodium

Spicy Edamame

Makes 4 servings

Prep Time: 5 minutes | Total Time: 15 minutes

3½ cups shelled edamame, fresh or frozen

2 teaspoons olive oil

2 teaspoons chili powder

1 teaspoon dried basil

½ teaspoon cumin

½ teaspoon black pepper

1. Preheat the oven to 375°F. Coat 2 baking sheets with cooking spray. In a bowl, combine the edamame, oil, chili powder, basil, cumin, and pepper. Spread the mixture over the baking sheets and coat with cooking spray.

2. Bake for 10 minutes, stirring once, or until the beans begin to brown.

3. Serve warm or chill to serve cold.

Per serving: 201 calories, 18 g protein, 13 g carbohydrates, 9 g total fat, 0.5 g saturated fat, 8 g fiber, 23 mg sodium

Egg Salad

Makes 4 servings

Prep Time: 15 minutes | Total Time: 25 minutes

8 eggs

¼ cup 0% plain Greek yogurt

5 green olives, chopped

2 ribs celery, chopped

2 teaspoons lemon juice

2 teaspoons capers

2 medium cucumbers, sliced

40 baby carrots

1. Place the eggs in a pot and cover with cool water about 1" higher than the eggs. Bring to a boil and boil for 1 minute. Remove from the heat, cover, and let stand for 10 minutes.

2. Meanwhile, prepare a bowl of ice water. Remove the eggs and immediately place in the ice water. Leave in the ice water for 3 minutes.

3. Crack and peel each egg and place in a mixing bowl. Add the yogurt, olives, celery, lemon juice, and capers and mash with a fork until just blended.

4. Divide the mixture among 4 bowls and surround each with one-quarter of the cucumber slices and 10 baby carrots.

Per serving: 207 calories, 16 g protein, 13 g carbohydrates, 11 g total fat, 3.5 g saturated fat, 4 g fiber, 338 mg sodium

Stuffed Sweet Potato Skins

Makes 4 servings
(6 potato wedges each)

Prep Time: 15 minutes | Total Time: 1 hour 15 minutes
plus cooling time

3 large sweet potatoes

⅔ cup grated Parmesan cheese

1 tablespoon chopped fresh parsley

1 teaspoon dried basil

½ teaspoon garlic powder

1 cup 0% plain Greek yogurt

2 tablespoons chopped scallions

1. Preheat the oven to 425°F. Line a baking sheet with foil. Pierce the potatoes a few times with a fork. Place on the prepared baking sheet. Bake for 1 hour, or until easily pierced with a fork. Remove and allow to cool for 15 minutes.

2. In a small bowl, combine the cheese, parsley, basil, and garlic powder.

3. Quarter the potatoes lengthwise. Scoop out the flesh (save for another meal), creating a ¼"-thick shell. Cut the strips in half crosswise, making 24 wedges. Place on a baking sheet. Coat both sides of the potatoes with cooking spray. Sprinkle with the cheese mixture.

4. Bake for 10 minutes, or until golden brown. To serve, top each wedge with 2 teaspoons of yogurt. Sprinkle with the scallions.

Per serving: 230 calories, 15 g protein, 32 g carbohydrates, 5 g total fat, 3 g saturated fat, 5 g fiber, 331 mg sodium

Tea Sandwiches

Makes 1 serving

Prep Time: 5 minutes | Total Time: 5 minutes

2 slices whole wheat bread, crusts cut off

1 tablespoon + 1 teaspoon reduced-fat cream cheese

1½ ounces reduced-sodium ham

⅛ medium cucumber, peeled and thinly sliced

1. Spread each slice of bread with 2 teaspoons of the cream cheese. Top one slice with the ham and cucumber slices. Top with the second slice of bread.

2. Cut bread in half and then horizontally in half again to make 4 small sandwiches total.

Per serving: 227 calories, 16 g protein, 25 g carbohydrates, 7 g total fat, 3 g saturated fat, 4 g fiber, 602 mg sodium

Sweet and Crunchy Greek Yogurt

Makes 1 serving

Prep Time: 5 minutes | Total Time: 5 minutes

1 cup 0% plain Greek yogurt

1½ tablespoons brown sugar

3 tablespoons high-fiber cereal

1. In a small bowl, combine yogurt and brown sugar.

2. Top with the cereal.

Per serving: 234 calories, 21 g protein, 39 g carbohydrates, 0.5 g total fat, 0 g saturated fat, 3 g fiber, 113 mg sodium

Chocolate Chip Cannoli

Makes 4 servings

Prep Time: 10 minutes | Total Time: 15 minutes plus cooling time

Butter-flavored cooking spray

4 whole wheat 96% fat-free flour tortillas (8″ diameter)

2 cups fat-free ricotta cheese

2 tablespoons confectioners' sugar

½ teaspoon vanilla extract

2 tablespoons mini chocolate chips

1. Preheat the oven to 250°F. Coat a baking sheet with cooking spray. Coat each tortilla with butter-flavored cooking spray on both sides, especially around the edges. Roll up each tortilla, overlapping the ends a bit, and place seam side down on the prepared baking sheet.

2. Bake for 5 minutes, or until the tortillas keep their shape. Place on a wire rack to cool.

3. In a medium bowl, with an electric mixer on medium speed, beat the ricotta cheese, sugar, and vanilla for 2 minutes, or until smooth. Stir in the chocolate chips.

4. To assemble, divide the filling among the cooled cannoli shells.

Per serving: 211 calories, 15 g protein, 30 g carbohydrates, 3 g total fat, 1.5 g saturated fat, 2 g fiber, 194 mg sodium

Cinnamon Swirl Yogurt

Makes 1 serving

Prep Time: 5 minutes | Total Time: 5 minutes

1 cup 0% plain Greek yogurt

1 teaspoon brown sugar

½ teaspoon ground cinnamon

½ teaspoon nutmeg

¼ teaspoon vanilla extract

2 tablespoons high-fiber cereal

1. In a small bowl, stir together the yogurt, sugar, cinnamon, nutmeg, and vanilla.

2. Top with the cereal.

Per serving: 173 calories, 21 g protein, 22 g carbohydrates, 1 g total fat, 0.5 g saturated fat, 3 g fiber, 102 mg sodium

Chocolate Raspberry Frozen Yogurt Pops

Makes 4 servings

Prep Time: 35 minutes | Total Time: 35 minutes plus freezing time

3 cups 0% plain Greek yogurt

2 cups fat-free milk

1 cup unsweetened frozen raspberries

¼ cup chocolate syrup

½ teaspoon vanilla extract

4 paper cups (16 ounces each)

4 frozen-pop sticks

1. In a blender, combine the yogurt, milk, raspberries, syrup, and vanilla. Blend for 2 minutes, scraping the sides of the blender as needed.

2. Arrange the paper cups in a 8" square pan. Divide the yogurt mixture among the cups. Freeze for 30 minutes. Insert a stick into each cup. Freeze for 1 hour, or until solid.

Per serving: 200 calories, 20 g protein, 29 g carbohydrates, 0 g total fat, 0.5 g saturated fat, 2 g fiber, 129 mg sodium

Minty Honey Frozen Treat

Makes 4 servings

Prep Time: 5 minutes | Total Time: 5 minutes plus freezing time

4 cups 0% plain Greek yogurt

¼ cup honey

2 tablespoons chopped spearmint leaves

1 tablespoon lemon juice

1 cup fresh or frozen unsweetened blackberries

1 cup fresh or frozen unsweetened raspberries

1. In a large stainless steel bowl, gently stir together the yogurt, honey, spearmint, and lemon juice.

2. Freeze for 2 hours, or until set.

3. Divide the mixture among 4 serving bowls. Top each portion with ½ cup berries.

Per serving: 218 calories, 21 g protein, 34 g carbohydrates, 0 g total fat, 0 g saturated fat, 4 g fiber, 87 mg sodium

Logging for Success

If you're aiming to lose weight, keeping track of what you eat throughout the day—whether on paper, on your Smartphone, or by using an online program such as the free My Health Trackers tool at www.prevention.com—helps to keep your calorie counts honest and helps you avoid those "forgotten" bites that can add up over the course of the day.

Just like with exercise, numerous studies have confirmed that dieters who keep track of what they eat are more likely to stay on target with their dieting goals. In one 14-week study from Bowling Green State University, a full 25 percent of the differences in how much weight different subjects lost was credited to whether or not they consistently kept track of what they ate. After all, having to admit to those cheese puffs on paper might make you think twice about whether you really want to eat them. In fact, those who lost more than 5 percent of their body weight on the program filled out logs on more than twice as many days as those who didn't lose at least 5 percent of their weight.

The sample log on the next page offers a good template to follow. Flip to page 309 in the Tone Every Inch Logs for a blank form you can photocopy.

Daily Food Log

Week of program: 2 **Date:** 3/11/12

MEAL	FOOD/ BEVERAGE CONSUMED	CALORIES/ PROTEIN/ FIBER	TIME OF DAY	OBSERVATIONS/ CHALLENGES
Breakfast	Cinnamon Pecan Oatmeal	432/27/10	7 a.m. preworkout Breakaway/ 8 a.m. ate the rest	Felt way less sluggish than usual after having the apple and yogurt before my workout.
Lunch	Turkey and Sprouts with Dill Spread and chips	370/24/12	12:15 p.m.	
Snack	1 Choc. Raspberry Frozen Yogurt Pop	200/20/2	4 p.m.	Hid a couple of these in the office freezer. Perfect afternoon pick-me-up!
Dinner	1 serving Lime Cilantro Black Beans	399/21/20	7 p.m.	No meat and my family actually liked it!
Optional Extra Snack				

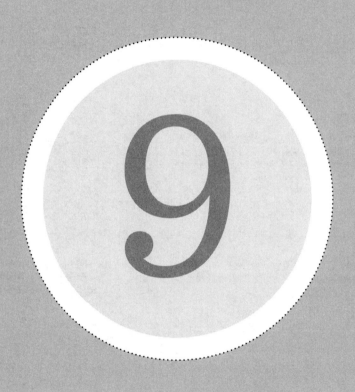

Overcoming Obstacles

We all have excuses for not working out. In fact, it often feels a lot easier to come up with an excuse than to lace up your sneakers or grab your dumbbells (until you get started, at least). That probably has a little something to do with the fact that to this day only about 16 percent of women actually meet the government's exercise guidelines. Heck, even I can come up with excuses, and exercise is in my job description!

Not only can our busy schedules make it seem hard to fit in workouts, but even with the best of intentions, the unexpected things that pop up (sick kids, a project that took longer than you expected, after-work happy hour with the colleague you've been dying to impress) can derail your plans. Then there's soreness, illness, injuries, and flat-out fatigue that can make it tempting (or even wise) to take a day (or several) off.

Especially if you joined this program after a long hiatus from any sort of strength training, I'll be the first to tell you that you are probably going to feel it at times—especially in the first couple of weeks as your body adjusts. In this chapter, I'm going to talk about some of the most common obstacles I've heard both from *Prevention* magazine readers

BEFORE YOU START

Taking a few simple steps to prepare before you launch into this body-sculpting adventure can help to seal your success.

Get (a) physical. Getting a doctor's checkup is something we should all be doing regularly, and it's an especially good idea before starting a new exercise program. A one-on-one with your GP can help to make sure you're setting smart goals for yourself and make you aware of any health risks that might affect your workouts. But that's not the only reason to make an appointment. Measuring your weight, cholesterol levels, blood pressure, and other health measures at the outset spells an extra motivational boost when you start to see those numbers improve. In a study by researchers at Texas A&M International University, volunteers who had a checkup before and after the winter holidays managed to stave off weight gain despite eating as much as one-third more calories thanks to ever-present seasonal goodies. Magic? More likely the awareness that they had a doc to report back to served as a push to squeeze in more activity.

and from the intrepid test panelists who served as this program's guinea pigs, and offer some suggestions to help you get through.

Brain Barriers

Perhaps the biggest thing to stand between you and your would-be workouts is your brain. That's right, you may think it's the junky weather, or your interminable to-do list, but at the end of the day, your brain's the boss and you decide what gets checked off the list and what doesn't. Luckily, psychologists are on the case, trying to figure out what makes us—and our workouts—tick. Here are a few mental tweaks that can help get you out the door.

Spread the word. Tell your husband, your kids, your co-workers, your best friend, and even your next-door neighbor about your plan to get in shape. Tempted to wait till the pounds come off to boast about your progress? Letting others in on your plan will both make you more accountable and give them the chance to pitch in with support when you need it, such as planning a carpool trade-off that allows you to sneak in morning workouts a couple days a week.

Write down your goals. The best (read: most likely to help you accomplish them) goals are best remembered by using the acronym SMART: specific, measurable, achievable, realistic, and time-based. Write down yours, keeping in mind that when it comes to weight loss, most experts agree that 1 to 2 pounds a week is a healthy amount to lose, while even ½ pound a week shows you're moving in the right direction. Write your goals on a sticky note and put it somewhere you'll see it often, like the corner of your computer screen or the bathroom mirror.

Bring an "I Think I Can" Attitude

Although obstacles are inevitable (hey, life happens!), research shows that the number one difference between those who overcome them to start and stick with exercising and those who don't is something psychologists call self-efficacy or, in other words, a can-do attitude. It's not about the size of the boulder in your way; it's about being the little engine that could. Put simply, the belief that you'll be able to overcome what life throws in your way—and planning for it—makes you more likely to become an exerciser for life.

Boost your odds by putting it on paper. List the barriers you know you're most likely to face over the course of this program (say, your husband unexpectedly having to work late and leaving you with the kids, or snow making it difficult to walk outside). Then brainstorm what you can do to stick with it when those things arise: exercising in the morning before things can get in the way (or lining up a neighborhood babysitter who's willing to come on short notice), and finding an indoor walking location such as a mall (or investing in a good cold-weather walking outfit).

Put Exercise First

Putting off your workout until the end of the day doesn't just make it more likely to fall off the end of your to-do list; it also may mean a lesser workout. That's because brain drain wears your body out, too. When Welsh researchers had subjects exercise after taking a mentally difficult test, they ran out of steam 15 percent faster than those who exercised after watching a video instead of taking the test. Another bonus: An impressive 75 percent of morning exercisers stick to their workouts, according to research from the Mollen Clinic in Scottsdale, Arizona.

Find the Right Motivation

While shedding pounds might top your list of goals for this program, looking a little deeper might make you more likely to stick with it to the finish (and achieve better results, weight loss included). In a study presented at the annual meeting of the American Council on Sports Medicine, would-be first-time marathoners who were focused on intrinsic goals like feeling good about the achievement were 70 percent more likely to cross the finish line than those who focused on losing weight or impressing others.

Time: The Ultimate Limited Resource

Lack of time is the most common excuse women give for skipping exercise. Between family and work, carpool and dishes, and for some of us, starting to care for an aging parent on top of it all, time can feel like the ultimate limited resource—and one you're helpless to change, at that. It's true, you can't stop the clock from ticking any more than you can

Helpful Hints: Make Over Your Motivation

Need an extra push to stick with your routine? Put your money where your mouth is. In a study from the Philadelphia Veterans Affairs Medical Center, folks who put up cold hard cash as collateral for hitting their weight loss goals were five times more likely to hit their mark—about half reached their goal, compared with only 10 percent of dieters who didn't have a cash incentive. I spoke to study author Leslie John, PhD, to better understand why money is such a big motivator. It turns out there are a couple of mind games at play. For one thing, we tend to be pretty cocky about our ability to lose weight when we start a new program, which makes us confident gamblers. And once the money is on the table, it hurts more to lose that cash than it feels good to not lose it (or even win money). The Web site stikk.com is a free forum where you can place a cash wager on your bet—and hopefully seal your success.

convince the car to go get its own oil change. But as busy as you are, I guarantee there are extra minutes hiding in your day that you could use more effectively if you knew how to pinpoint them. So put on your detective hat and let's get started.

➲ Helpful Hints: Check Your Tech

If you're a mom, you've probably uttered some version of the words "No more (insert: TV/Internet/texting) until you've (insert: cleaned your room/finished your homework/eaten a civilized dinner)." Well, it's time to turn that same tough love on yourself. All the technology that's supposed to make us more efficient can turn into one big procrastination party, allowing passive distractions to eat into time that could be used to do something you *choose* to do (like exercise!). If we let ourselves respond to every *ding* of the inbox or peek at Facebook whenever temptation flits by, that is. But some helpful online tools can serve to illuminate just how your online habits might be extending your workday (while getting *less* done), and even put the kibosh on temptation. Here are three to try.

Find out what you really do. RescueTime (www.rescuetime.com) tracks your time spent on different Web sites and apps, and with the Pro version ($6/month) even particular documents, and churns out graphs revealing just how much time you fritter away online shopping.

Say sayonara to temptation. Like parental controls for your time, adding LeechBlock (addons.mozilla.org) to your Firefox Web browser lets you ban certain time-sucking sites during certain hours, or impose limits, such as no more than 10 minutes a day on Facebook.

Take a Web time-out. If your job doesn't actually require you to be online, cutting off your Internet access could help you boost productivity big time. Don't have the self-control? For $10, Macfreedom (www.macfreedom.com) will do it for you, blocking Web connectivity for up to 8 hours at a time.

Do a Time Inventory

Take 2 days (starting now!) and keep track of exactly how you spend your time. It turns out that Americans have nearly twice as much downtime as we think we do, according to a poll by Harris Interactive. Often this extra time is hidden in chunks through the day, making it easy to miss, but writing it down helps you to see time sucks for what they are.

Settle for Imperfect

Women are notorious perfectionists. "You just have to prioritize sometimes," says Jessica Smith, a personal trainer and certified wellness coach in Miami. "Look at the house and say, 'Maybe the house isn't perfect today, but I'm going to get my workout in.'"

Quit Multitasking

Think you're a master at doing three things at once? Scientists beg to differ. And the more you do it, the worse at multitasking you likely are, say Stanford University researchers who found that heavy multitaskers had more difficulty filtering out distractions and were slower at switching between different tasks. A collaboration between Microsoft and researchers at the University of Illinois studied actual workers' computer activity over 2 weeks to see how much of a slowdown actually occurred when people stopped what they were doing to check e-mail or respond to an instant chat message. It turns out e-mail breaks averaged 10 minutes, while chat conversations pulled workers away from the project they were working on for an average of 8 minutes a pop. Turn off new message alerts and you might just find you have time for a workout.

Fill Your Empty Pockets of Time

You might think finding a spare 10 minutes in your day is more like finding a nickel in your pocket than a $20 bill. But the women who test-drove this program would beg to differ. For Merry Buckley, who lost 11 pounds on the program (and has kept on losing since), this routine worked because of its ability to fit into the cracks in her day. "Having something to do while I'm also watching the kids or getting dinner started or cycling the laundry really helps," she says. "It's not like running, where I have to have a block of time with no responsibilities for a half hour or an hour. It can be broken up into the time I have."

Katrina Walker also learned that even a consistent 10 or 15 minutes a day could make a difference of several inches around her waist and hips as well as big strength gains. "I didn't like doing two full 30-minute sessions a week, but I found if I did a shorter routine of 15 minutes in the morning more like 5 times a week, it worked well for me," she says. "And if I can only get two-thirds of the routine done in the morning, now I come home and know I only have a few more minutes to finish up in the evening." The bottom line: Every little bit counts.

The Common "Ouch"

Working out doesn't have to hurt to do your body good. But the reality is, some aches and pains often come with the package, whether it's next-day soreness after a tough workout or, worse, a muscle pull or other injury. While there's no one-size-fits-all prescription for relief (and any serious or ongoing pain should be discussed with your doctor), here are some tips to overcome common physical ailments you might run into on this or any workout plan.

Soreness Do's and Don'ts

Ah, it hurts so good (just keep telling yourself that). While sharp or shooting pain usually signals an injury worth listening to, feeling more general body soreness a day or two after a tough workout is perfectly healthy. Here's how getting stronger works: When you push your body to do something it's not used to, like use an 8-pound dumbbell for an arm exercise you used to do with a 5-pounder, the extra push actually damages your muscle, creating little microtears. But don't worry—that's not a bad thing. The healing process that follows is what leaves your muscle stronger and more toned than when you began. Unfortunately, nothing but time can heal those soreness-inducing tears, but there are some things you can do to feel better in the meantime.

Do: Drink milk. Refueling ASAP after your workout with a combination of carbohydrates (to restock your muscles' stores) and protein (to help muscles heal and grow) has long been accepted as the best way to avoid energy dips later in the day and make sure you're on top of your game for tomorrow's workout. Now a series of studies have suggested that milk—specifically chocolate milk—might be the best choice, thanks to an ideal protein and carbohydrate blend that muscles can slurp up and use quickly to rejuvenate. Turns out sipping the white stuff (or its chocolaty cousin) after a strength workout might help to reduce muscle soreness over the subsequent 48 hours, perhaps because it seems to spur more rebuilding of muscles, say scientists at Northumbria University in Newcastle, England.

Don't: Get in the hot tub. It may sound soothing, but hot water can actually increase inflammation and soreness in already-compromised muscles—and this goes for the heat brought on by any hot bath, hot tub, or even saunas and steam rooms. However, if you can't resist the tub, toss in some Epsom salt (available at drugstores), which some believe helps reduce inflammation and pain.

Do: Bring on the ice. A bag of frozen peas can do wonders for easing inflammation and soreness, but for ultimate relief (after the initial shock) try an ice bath. A common trick of elite athletes, dumping a bag (or a couple trays) of ice into a bathtub filled with cold water can help to minimize soreness. The cold causes your blood vessels to constrict, which limits the increase in bloodflow to the damaged muscles initially (like kinking a hose). Then, when you get out of the cold tub and warm up, the blood gushes through with healing nutrients, helping to flush out some of the soreness-causing agents in the blood, explains Greg Ranalli, an athletic trainer in Wayne, Pennsylvania, who has published several studies on the effects of body cooling for athletes. Still prefer to sip your ice water, not sit in it? Try a cool shower instead of a hot one.

Don't: Stretch (too much). While some light stretching feels good on sore muscles thanks to what some experts describe as an analgesic effect, overdoing it could actually do more damage than good and even prolong your recovery, says David Geier, MD, an orthopedic surgeon and the director of sports medicine at the Medical University of South Carolina in Charleston.

Do: Pop an anti-inflammatory. If you want to, that is. NSAIDs, including ibuprofen (Advil), acetaminophen (Tylenol), and naproxen (Aleve), can help to ease soreness and inflammation, as well as lower levels of an enzyme that signals muscle damage. They can help you feel better, but they won't get you back to your A-game any faster than simply waiting it out. If you are going to pop pills, stick to the recommended dosage on the bottle, and keep taking them as recommended for a couple of days. Take 'em just once and you won't realize the inflammation-squelching benefits.

Do: Get a massage (or give yourself one). While research is mixed, a good rubdown has been shown to reduce swelling and lessen soreness by as much as 30 percent, and we're willing to take these odds. While an hour-long professional session is great if you have the time and the bucks to pay for it, studies suggest as little as 10 minutes on a sore muscle can do the trick. If you can't get to a pro, a DIY leg massage is wholly within your (or your husband's) talents: Alternate between gliding palms over the length of the muscle, kneading in small circles, and drumming up and down the length of the muscle to increase healing bloodflow.

Injury 101

The best-laid get-fit plan can be derailed quickly if you refuse to listen to your body when it needs a break. But most injuries can be nipped in the bud if you catch them early and proceed with caution.

MUSCLE PULLS

What it is: A sudden pain that happens midworkout, usually as a result of going past the range of motion your body is ready for (for example, taking off at a sprint without warming up enough).

Prevent it: Warm up thoroughly by going through the same sorts of movements you'll be doing when you take your workout to full speed. For cardio like walking or running, starting slow and gradually increasing the pace of your walk or run will do the trick. For strength training, if you're planning to exercise your arms, you'll need to get those going, too. This gets extra blood pumping to the parts of your body that are moving and lubricates the joints so they can move smoothly through a healthy range of motion.

Fix it: Rest and ice are your two best tools. Depending on what muscle you pulled, you may be able to keep up with exercises that don't aggravate it. For example, I strained my wrist while writing this book (a too-much-too-soon dose of gardening, not the workouts or the writing!). I was able to keep up with cardio workouts—including intervals—but I had to take a 1-week time-out on some of the strength exercises that were painful. Depending on how quickly you make the call, as little as a couple of days off might be all the healing you need (I stubbornly went back to the same activity that had aggravated my wrist for another day before I called it quits, hence my longer bench time). For icing to reduce inflammation and ease soreness, refreezeable gel packs are great to have on hand, but a bag of frozen veggies works, too. Simply hold it on the painful area for about 15 minutes a couple of times a day with plenty of warmup time between bouts.

BACK PAIN

What it is: Triggered by anything from chronic poor posture and weak core muscles to acute muscle strains, pain is most common in the lower back because most of your body weight is supported there.

Prevent it: The exercises (strength and cardio) on this plan are actually a great start at preventing back pain. Despite the now-outdated popular belief, rest is not always best for back pain since the boost in bloodflow you get from exercise is incredibly beneficial for bad backs. And some studies suggest that strength training might be even better than cardio because it involves the whole body rather than just the legs like many aerobic workouts do. Beyond that, focused core stability exercise such as Pilates has been a proven back-saver, and main-

WHEN TO SEE A DOCTOR

Although most of the injuries discussed in this section will usually go away on their own given enough R&R (as well as ice and ibuprofen), knowing when it's time to call the doctor can help you avoid prolonging (or worse, aggravating) an injury that needs expert attention. There are unfortunately no hard-and-fast rules for when to get to the doctor's office, but David Geier, MD, an orthopedic surgeon and the director of sports medicine at the Medical University of South Carolina in Charleston, offers these guidelines.

It happened suddenly. Turning an ankle usually falls into the category of "gets better on its own." A torn ligament in your knee, on the other hand, might require surgery and could get worse if you don't get treatment. If it happened suddenly, and the pain is excruciating, it's probably worth the copay to get it checked out.

It's not getting better. "Your injury doesn't have to be completely healed within a week or two," says Dr. Geier, "but if it hasn't improved at all by then, it's a good idea to see someone."

It's limiting your ability to live your life. If the pain is so severe that you can't get around, work, or do what you need to do, a physician can help you determine the best course of action to speed your recovery.

You notice these warning signs. Shooting pain, numbness, tingling, weakness in a limb, or catching in a joint (like your knee) can all be warning signs of a more severe injury.

taining healthy flexibility can help, too (see the stretching routine on page 180).

Fix it: Let pain be your guide on this. If walking feels okay but the increased impact of running is no good, stick to walking. If neither of those are pain free, swimming might be a good option. If you're completely out of commission, a few days of rest might be in order, but when you are able to get moving again, do what feels good.

IT BAND FRICTION SYNDROME

What it is: This is typically felt as a pain in the knee, though it's often traced back to weakness in the glute muscles (aka the butt) and subsequent tightness in the iliotibial band, which is a band of connective tissue running up the side of your leg connecting the knee to the hip.

Prevent it: This program is a great start (the Butt Kicker and Side Leg-Lift Crunch are both variations on exercises often prescribed to help with runner's knee because they're very targeted glute exercises). Regular stretching can also help. One to add: Sit in a chair, left foot on the floor, and cross your right leg over, resting your right ankle on your left knee. Hold for up to 30 seconds at a time, making sure to stretch both sides.

Fix it: Ice, ice, baby. But remember, even if your knee is the spot that hurts, the whole length of your thigh is involved. I like to freeze a cup of ice and rub it up and down the length of the side of my leg to combine ice with a massage for the tight area. Some experts also swear by foam rollers, which you can roll under your leg, using the weight of your body to press into the area. And above all, this is an injury that's best to nip in the bud, because trying to push through can create a frustrating cycle of inflammation and pain. Let discomfort be your guide, but runner's knee shouldn't prevent you from doing most of the strength exercises on this plan, and some experimentation should help you to find a type of cardio that doesn't bother it. Swimming is a great one to try, for example, because it doesn't involve any bending of the knee.

SHIN SPLINTS

What it is: Pain or burning running up the front of your lower leg when you walk or run.

Prevent it: The top cause of shin splints is increasing your workout too quickly. Another culprit: spent shoes. Make sure to replace your walking or running shoes after covering 300 to 500 miles in them (or every 150 hours of workout wear).

Fix it: While the burning sensation in your shins can be uncomfortable, this isn't typically a diagnosis that means stopping altogether. Stretching your calves thoroughly (see page 184) as well as strengthening the tiny muscles that surround the shin and are used to control ankle movement can help. Try these exercises.

○ **Heel rockers:** Rock back onto your heels with your toes up as high as you can lift them, then up onto your toes. Repeat up to 20 times.

○ **Heel walks:** Walk on your heels with your toes lifted for about 20 steps. Now do it again, this time with your toes up and pointing out to the sides. Walk a third time on your heels, toes pointing in toward each other. Yes, it looks silly, but this will work the stabilizer muscles from every angle.

PLANTAR FASCIITIS

What it is: This catchall term for arch pain refers to the connective tissue you can feel under your arch that runs from the ball of your big toe all the way to the base of your calf muscle. The pain is usually felt just behind the ball of your toe, but it often stems from a shortened calf muscle, making stretching the calf key to prevention.

Prevent it: Because high heels put the calf in a shortened position, wearing flats can help.

Fix it: Hide your stilettos, for starters! Stretch your calf morning, noon, and night, and ice the arch area several times a day. Typically the pain will be strongest first thing in the morning and will loosen up over the course of the day, so shifting your workouts to the p.m. may help. If weight-bearing exercises like walking and running bother it too much, switching to biking, swimming, or lower-impact elliptical may help.

CELEBRATING THE POSITIVES

Don't focus on the bad things that could derail your progress on this plan. One of the best ways to stay motivated to stick with a healthy new lifestyle like this one is to stop and celebrate the small steps. Maybe it's doing all the scheduled workouts 1 week without skipping any, or losing your first 5 pounds. Giving yourself a fun treat helps to ensure all of your hard work and willpower don't go unnoticed. Here are 10 ideas—big and little—to get you started.

O Go shopping for a cute (and flattering!) new workout outfit.

O Take time out for a coffee date with a friend you rarely have time to catch up with.

O Get a massage.

O Take a bubble bath.

O Get your makeup done.

O Hire professional cleaners to come to your house.

O Go to the movies.

O Put your husband and kids in charge of giving you one breakfast in bed.

O Read a good book.

O Plan a day trip to explore a state park you've never visited.

Katrina Walker

Age 47

Lost: 4 inches from her waist and hips

Gained: The discipline to stick with a workout routine for the first time

Favorite workout: Fat Blast Minute Intervals combining hiking and running with her dogs

A pair of energetic rescue dogs kept Katrina Walker, 47, active with regular hiking on the trails around her hometown, but she'd never managed to make strength training a habit she could stick with. And with high risk for osteoporosis, depression, and colon and breast cancer running in her family, she knew how important a well-rounded program of cardio and strength was for staying healthy. The goal: to get better at self-discipline and talking herself into working out by focusing on the reasons *to* do it rather than reasons not to.

After completing the 8-week Tone Every Inch test panel, Katrina's hiking legs are nearly 15 percent stronger than when she started—a helpful boost for chasing down the more youthful of her two dogs, Dexter, when he tries to take off without her across the parking lot at the trailhead.

She's also shaved off more than 2.5 inches from her waist and nearly 1.5 in her hips, which translates to better-fitting pants. "I feel better in my clothes," she says. "Less stiff and lighter, as though I've shed an extra layer."

But the biggest achievement for Katrina is in her head. "I feel better mentally about the fact that I'm sticking with an exercise regimen," she says. "This morning I didn't have time to do my full workout, so I just did two-thirds of it. I came home today and I was like, 'Well, I just have a couple more minutes' and I just did it whereas in the past I wouldn't have. I would have been like, 'Oh, heck with it. I'll do it tomorrow.' But now I have a habit, and even if I screw it up, I'm more likely to get back on task with it."

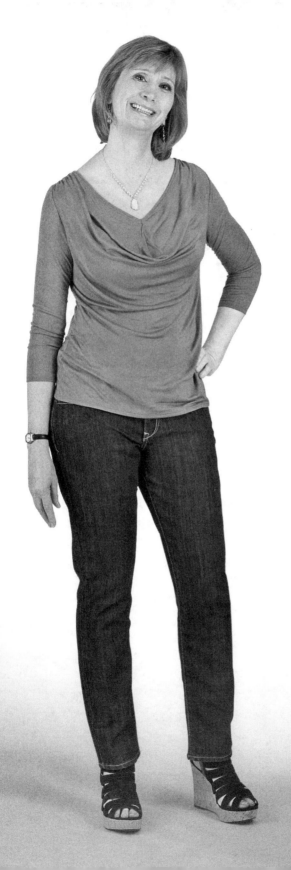

271

10

I Did It! What Now?

Congratulations! Before we go any further, I want you to give yourself a big pat on the back. Chances are you had your bumps along the way—our testers persevered through sick kids, muscle injuries, and even military deployment—but you made it to 8 weeks and that's an accomplishment. Think back to that first week. Did your legs wobble as you tried to figure out the exercises? Whether or not you've made it to your weight loss goal, you should be feeling lighter, tighter, and more energized.

So what now? Well, I hope these past 8 weeks have taught you just how good exercise can make you feel (even when it makes you feel a bit sore!). In fact, the longer you stick with regular exercise, the bigger feel-good boost it gives you, according to researchers at the Sacramento, California, VA Medical Center. While just one workout can lift your spirits, the study found that mood benefits doubled after 6 months. Which is good, because we're just getting started! The next step is to revisit your goals, appreciate what you've accomplished to this point, and then decide what your goal will be for the next 8 weeks. This chapter will help you to choose your next goal and then decide on a plan for success.

Option 1: Tone Every Inch 2.0

Choose this if: You're loving the program so far and want to know how to take it to the next level (but you'd rather do so without having to learn new moves!).

The Tone Every Inch plan is designed to be adaptable for readers with a wide range of abilities and backgrounds. If you're happy with the program and the results you've been seeing so far, there's no reason you can't keep it going. But to make sure you keep seeing those great results and steer clear of dreaded plateaus, we're going to give the 8 weeks a slightly different spin this time.

Cardio 2.0

Continue to do the Intensity Cardio workouts in Chapter 5, aiming for at least two and up to three per week. If you have time, add some moderate sessions and consider making one workout per week longer—up to an hour.

Don't forget: As you get fitter and stronger, you'll be able to maintain a faster pace with less effort. Good news, but it means you either need to speed up or keep it up longer to get the same results. Use how you feel as a guide, remembering that your definitions of the different RPE levels on page 107 will have changed since you began.

Strength 2.0

Continue to do at least two and up to three strength workouts a week. You'll still start with band-only exercises (this time for 4 weeks) and then switch to combo workouts for Weeks 5 through 8, but this time with a different twist.

In the first 8 weeks, the progression element was all about mastering the two sets of exercises and gradually increasing the amount of high-intensity cardio you could do. Now that you've successfully accomplished all that, to allow you to continue with the same exercises without allowing your body to get bored and plateau, we're going to introduce something called periodization. Periodization is a technique used by athletes to change up their training over the course of the year in order to perform at their best. At the root, this is done by alternating cycles that challenge the body in different ways, as well as cycles that are harder and easier, in order to give the body a rejuvenating break and avoid overtraining or injuries that can stall results. For Tone Every Inch 2.0, we're going to break the 8-week session into four 2-week cycles: recovery, speed, power, and strength. Here's how it works.

WEEKS 1 AND 2: RECOVERY (TWO STRENGTH WORKOUTS A WEEK)

You've just completed a challenging 8 weeks! Just like the recovery periods in your interval cardio workouts allow you to go harder and faster during the intervals, giving you a more effective workout than if you just pushed straight through, the same is true of resistance exercise. Giving your muscles an active-recovery break—still working them, but at a slightly lower intensity—will allow you to pick it up again in the next cycle with even more effective muscle-toning workouts.

For this 2-week cycle, do 12 to 15 repetitions of each of the 10 band exercises in Chapter 3. Make sure to use a band that fatigues your muscle by the end of the set.

In Week 1, do just one set. In Week 2, try to complete two sets of each exercise.

WEEKS 3 AND 4: BANDS ON SPEED
(TWO OR THREE STRENGTH WORKOUTS A WEEK)

While we focused on slow repetitions when we first learned these moves, there are some benefits to moving faster—especially with bands. For this 2-week cycle, do 15 to 20 repetitions of the 10 band exercises, moving as quickly as you can through the band-stretching portion of the move. At the top of the move (when the band is stretched to its fullest), pause before you release the resistance, then release slowly and with control.

Start with one set in Week 3, and increase to two sets in Week 4.

WEEKS 5 AND 6: TRIPLE-TONING POWER

In this cycle, you'll follow the same fast-on-the-way-up/slow-on-the-way-down technique you used in Weeks 3 and 4, but this time you'll add back the weights. Reduce your reps, aiming to complete 12 to 15 reps of each exercise and fatiguing your muscle by the final rep of each set.

Do one or two sets in Week 5, and increase to two or three sets in Week 6.

WEEKS 7 AND 8: TRIPLE-TONING STRENGTH

For this final cycle, we'll return to slow-controlled lifting on the up and the down portions of the exercises. Increase the size of the weight you're lifting, both because you should be feeling stronger by now and because the focus of this cycle is strength and you'll be doing fewer repetitions. Choose a weight one size up from what you usually use. If you can't complete all the reps (aim to do 5 to 8 reps of each exercise), simply set the dumbbell down and finish the set with only the band.

Do one or two sets in Week 7, and increase to two or three sets in Week 8.

Option 2: Tone Every Inch: Bonus Strength Workout

Choose this if: You're dying for some new moves to mix things up.

Switching up your exercises periodically is a great way to avoid boredom and plateaus. Even if two exercises target the same primary muscle group, if the movement or positioning is changed, you'll be working the muscle in a new way and likely engaging a different crew of smaller supporting muscles as well.

Start by doing one to three sets of 8 to 12 reps of the following eight exercises, using a dumbbell-and-band combo that fatigues you by the last rep in each set. Aim to do the entire routine two or three times a week. Once you get comfortable with the moves, if you're ready to switch it up again, you can experiment with the Tone Every Inch 2.0 plan starting on page 275.

Balancing Kickback

(feel it in your: triceps)

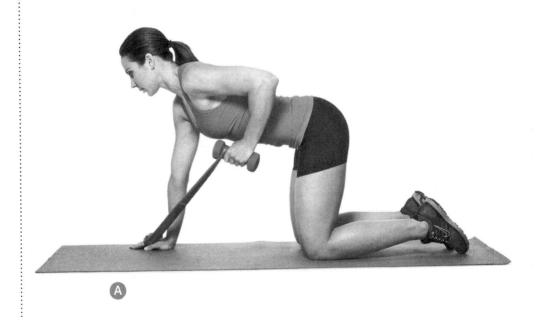

A

Step 1. Get into a tabletop position with your hands under your shoulders, knees under your hips, back straight, and abs pulled in, a band anchored near the floor in front of you. (If you don't have a door or a sturdy piece of furniture nearby, you can simply anchor the band by holding it with your support hand.)

Step 2. Pick up the free end of the band plus a dumbbell in your left hand, and bend your left elbow to about 90 degrees, with your upper arm along your side. The band should be taut (Photo A).

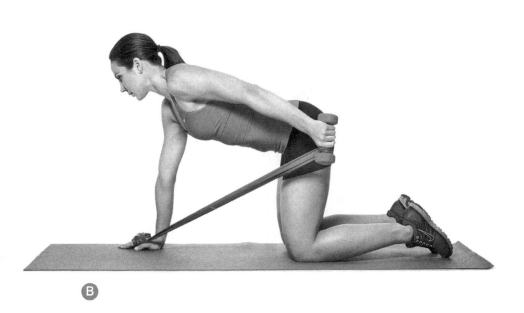

(B)

Step 3. Press the band and dumb-bell straight back (Photo B). Slowly lower back to start. Do 8 to 12 reps, then switch sides and repeat.

➡ *Make It Harder*
When pressing the band and dumbbell straight back, simultaneously extend your right leg straight back, squeezing your glutes.

Balancing Bent-Over Row

(feel it in your: back, arms, and glutes)

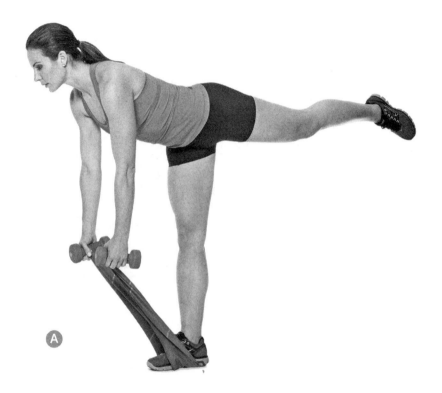

A

Step 1. Stagger your feet with your right foot in front. Place the middle of the band under your right foot, and grasp one end of the band along with a dumbbell in each hand.

Step 2. With your right knee slightly bent, hinge forward from your hips and extend your left leg straight back until your torso and left leg are about parallel to the floor, arms hanging straight down perpendicular to the floor (Photo A).

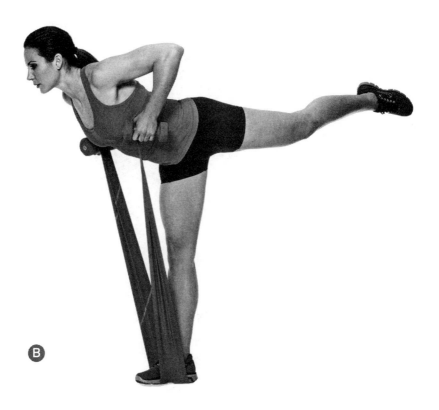

(B)

Step 3. Bend your elbows to pull the band and dumbbells up near your underarms (Photo B).

Step 4. Pulse the elevated leg up an inch or two, then lower your arms to the starting position. Do half a set (4 to 6 reps), then switch the balancing leg and do another 4 to 6 reps. Build up to doing an entire set on one leg, then doing a second set with the opposite leg.

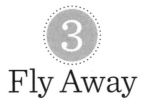

Fly Away

(feel it in your: shoulders)

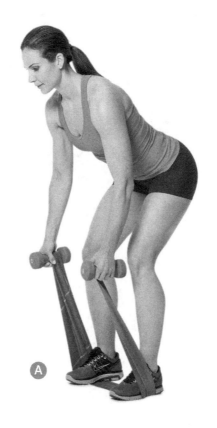

(A)

Step 1. Stand with your feet hip-width apart, a band under both feet with one end plus a dumbbell in each hand.

Step 2. Slightly bending your knees, hinge forward from your hips, back flat, until your torso is about parallel with the floor. Let your arms hang straight down perpendicular to the floor, with a slight bend in your elbows and your palms facing each other (Photo A).

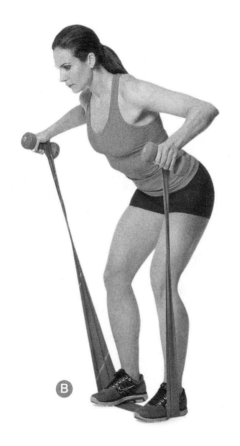

Step 3. Draw your elbows up and to the sides until they're at shoulder height (imagine you're a marionette doll with strings attached to your elbows only and pulling upward) (Photo B). Lower your arms back to the front. Repeat for 8 to 12 reps.

Squat and Lift

(feel it in your: shoulders, glutes, and thighs)

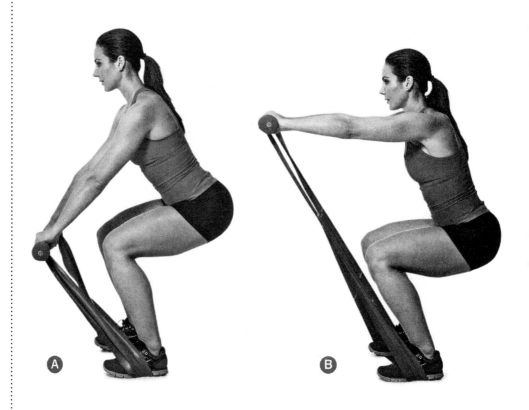

A

B

Step 1. Stand with your feet hip-width apart, the band under both feet with one end plus a dumbbell in each hand.

Step 2. Bend your knees and sit back as though into a chair (Photo A).

Step 3. Raise your arms straight to the front (Photo B).

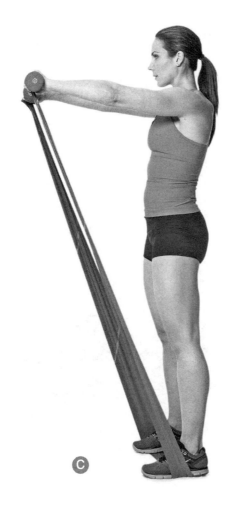

Step 4. Straighten your legs to stand (Photo C), then slowly lower your arms to the sides.

Step 5. Repeat, this time raising your arms straight out to the sides after you bend your knees to squat; stand, then lower your arms. Repeat for 8 to 12 reps to complete a set (each arm lift is 1 rep).

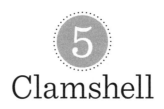

Clamshell

(feel it in your: glutes)

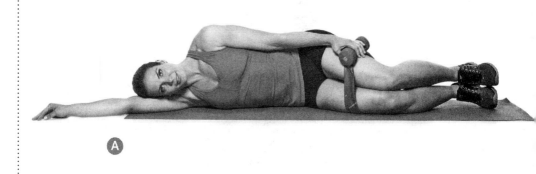

A

Step 1. Lie on your right side, legs stacked with knees bent about 90 degrees.

Step 2. Tie the resistance band in a secure loop just above your knees so it's snug but not stretched with legs together (Photo A).

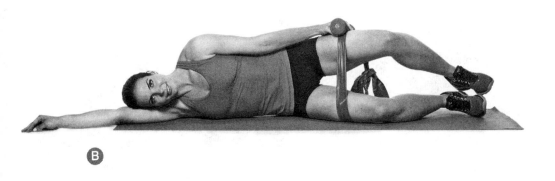

(B)

Step 3. Keeping your heels together, rotate your left hip up, opening your left knee away from your right, which remains stationary (Photo B). Pause, then lower to the starting position. Repeat for 8 to 12 reps, then switch sides to complete 1 set.

6

Chest Press Crunch

(feel it in your: abs, arms, and chest)

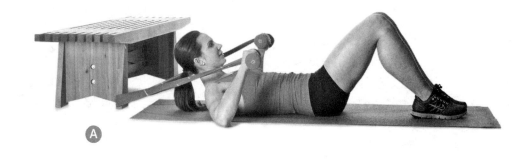

Ⓐ

Step 1. Anchor the middle of a band near the floor and lie in front of it with your knees bent, feet flat.

Step 2. Grasp one end of the band plus a dumbbell in each hand and bend your elbows to hold the band and dumbbells near your chest.

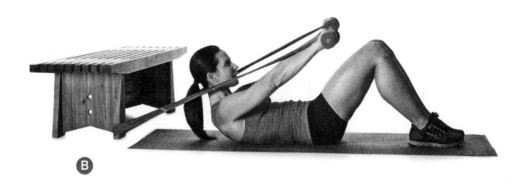

B

Step 3. Lift your upper back and shoulders off the floor into a crunch (Photo A).

Step 4. Without lowering your torso, straighten your elbows and press your arms diagonally forward and up, perpendicular to your body (Photo B). Now slowly lower your torso and arms back to the starting position. Do 8 to 12 reps to complete a set.

Scissor Press

(feel it in your: hips, thighs, and shoulders)

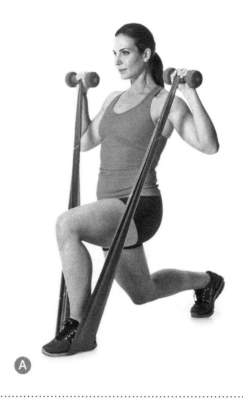

Ⓐ

Step 1. Stand in a split stance, your left foot about 2 to 3 feet in front of the right. Step on the center of the band with your left foot and hold an end in each hand, along with dumbbells, with elbows bent and dumbbells at shoulder height. (If your band is too short, use two and put one end of each band under the same foot, with the other end in each hand.)

Step 2. Bend both knees to lower into a lunge, left knee over ankle (Photo A).

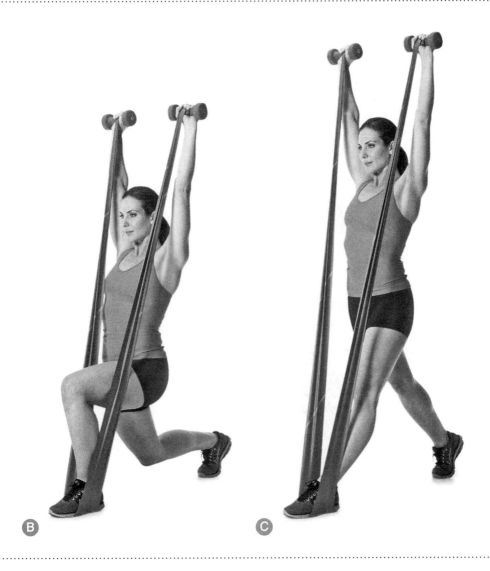

Step 3. Straighten your elbows to press the dumbbells overhead (Photo B).

Step 4. Stand first (Photo C), then lower your arms to the starting position. Do 8 to 12 reps, then switch sides to complete a set.

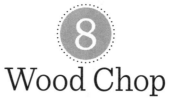

Wood Chop

(feel it in your: abs, glutes, and thighs)

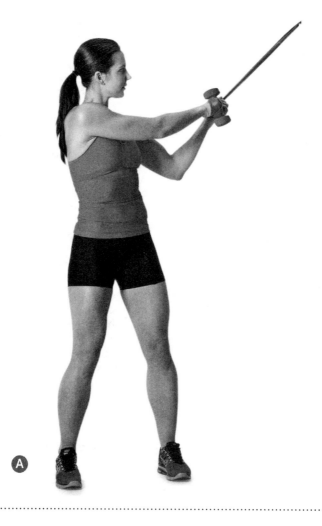

A

Step 1. Anchor the band overhead to your left side and hold the loose end of the band plus a dumbbell with both hands in front of you, reaching across your body toward the anchor (Photo A).

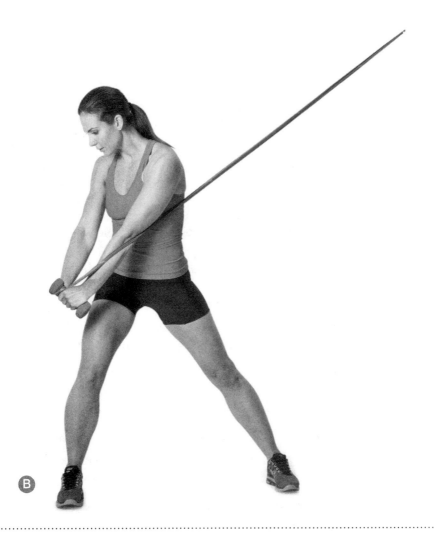

(B)

Step 2. Take a big step toward the right with your right foot, and bend your right knee into a side lunge (your left leg stays straight). Simultaneously pull the band down and across your body, rotating your torso toward the right (Photo B). Return to the starting position. Do 8 to 12 reps, then turn and repeat, pulling in the opposite direction.

Option 3: Tone Every Inch— Even Faster

Choose this if: You're lucky to get in four workouts a week (two strength and two cardio) and you want to do more with less.

If you want to trim down your workout time while still maintaining or continuing the toning and weight loss you've achieved this far, this is the workout plan for you. To minimize the number of workouts you have to do per week, we've added cardio intervals to the strength routine, giving you Intensity Cardio and strength all in one workout.

Aim to do the Triple-Toning Strength workout (see page 276) two or three times a week. After each strength exercise, do 30 to 60 seconds of your choice of the Fat Blast Interval options below. (You don't have to do the same one throughout the workout—mix and match to work your body in different ways.) For best results, add a dose of Moderate Cardio when you have time on alternate days throughout the week.

Fat Blast Interval Options

1. **Stair running:** If you have a flight of stairs where you're exercising, run up and down it as many times as you can in 30 seconds. Keep track, and challenge yourself to increase your number as you improve.

2. **Jumping jacks:** Back to boot camp—this is the old standard. Jump up, landing with your feet wide, arms overhead. Jump again, bringing feet together and arms down to your sides.

3. **Rope skipping:** If you have a jump rope, use it. If not, just pretend you're turning a rope and jumping forward and back over it.

4. **Line hops:** Place a piece of masking tape on the floor, or find a line you can keep your eye on (such as the edge of a tile). Feet together, hop side to side, back and forth over the line. For an added challenge, upgrade the line to a small object such as a water bottle that you have to jump up over.

5. **Ups and downs:** Feet wide, bend your knees and hinge forward from your hips to touch the ground with your fingertips. From

that position, jump up, reaching arms overhead. Land with knees soft, then touch the ground and jump again.

6. **Band pass:** Grab your band and bunch it up in your right hand. Lift your right knee as high as you can, and pass the band from your right to your left hand underneath your lifted leg. Lift your left leg and pass the band back. To keep it low impact, continue as a high-knee march. To bump it up a notch, add a hop on each foot as you raise the other knee.

Option 4: Tone Every Inch Turbocharged

Choose this if: You want more! You're willing to exercise an hour a day if it gets rid of the weight.

While you can certainly see phenomenal results from exercising as little as 20 to 30 minutes a day (something the testers of this plan can attest to), some studies do suggest that committing more time to exercise can help you take off more weight and keep it off for good. While there's no real benefit to doing more than the two to three strength workouts a week that you've already been doing, increasing the duration of your Intensity Cardio workouts is where you'll get the most bang for your buck. (For strength on this plan, follow the periodized plan outlined in Option 1.)

You can continue to do the Intensity Cardio routines in Chapter 5 two or three times per week, but starting this week, increase the length of your workouts by about 10 percent a week. For example, if your current workout length is 30 minutes, you should aim to increase it to 33 minutes the first week, then 36, then 40 and so on until you're doing between 45 and 60 minutes per workout. Think of the 10 percent as a rule of thumb—not an exact prescription. If you're doing the Fat Blast 30-Second Intervals, for example, it's okay to add one extra interval a week (4 minutes and 30 seconds, including the recovery) even though it's slightly more than 10 percent. To keep things interesting, here are a few more Intensity Cardio workouts to add to your repertoire.

Up and Down the Ladder

I love ladder intervals because they allow you to ease into a workout by gradually building up the length of the intervals. Then, on the way "down" the ladder at the end of the workout, you can really push yourself, knowing that each interval is shorter than the last.

Here's how it works: After warming up with 3 to 5 minutes at an easy pace of the activity you'll be doing for your workout, pick it up to a level 7 or 8 (see "Quick Guide to RPE" on page 107) for 1 minute. Slow down for a recovery of the same length as your interval. Add 1 minute to your interval duration (and accompanying recovery) until you get to 5 minutes. That's the top of the ladder. After you've done your 5-minute interval and 5-minute rest, start subtracting a minute from each interval until you're back to 1 minute. If you're just starting out, only go up to 4 minutes for a 40-minute workout, or 3 minutes for a 32-minute workout.

ACTIVITY	TIME	EFFORT LEVEL
Warmup	0:00–5:00	4–5
Interval 1	5:00–6:00	7–8
Recovery	6:00–7:00	5–6
Interval 2	7:00–9:00	7–8
Recovery	9:00–11:00	5–6
Interval 3	11:00–15:00	7–8
Recovery	15:00–18:00	5–6
Interval 4	18:00–22:00	7–8
Recovery	22:00–26:00	5–6
Interval 5	26:00–31:00	7–8
Recovery	31:00–36:00	5–6
Interval 6	36:00–40:00	7–8
Recovery	40:00–44:00	5–6
Interval 7	44:00–47:00	7–8
Recovery	47:00–50:00	5–6
Interval 8	50:00–52:00	7–8
Recovery	52:00–54:00	5–6
Interval 9	54:00–55:00	7–8
Recovery	55:00–56:00	5–6
Cooldown	56:00–58:00	4–5

It's All Downhill

Want to know what I like better than ladder workouts? Ones where you only have to do the downward part of the ladder! These workouts start with longer intervals that decrease in length as the workout progresses. While the always-shorter-than-the-last interval style can be mentally encouraging, it's also a great way to hone your speed skills. Early in the workout, when you're getting into the swing of things, the intervals are long enough to be challenging even if you're not running on all cylinders yet. But by the time you get to the end, you'll show off your speed.

Here's how it works: After warming up with 3 to 5 minutes at an easy pace of the activity you'll be doing for your workout, pick it up to a level 7 or 8 (see "Quick Guide to RPE" on page 107) for 8 minutes. Slow down for 2 minutes to recover, then increase your pace again, dropping 1 minute from each interval until you're down to 1. If you're just starting out and 50 minutes is too long, subtract one or two of the longer intervals. For example, if you skip the 7-minute interval, dropping from 8 to 6, you'll be left with a 41-minute routine. Eliminate the 5-minute interval (so you'll go 8, 6, 4, 3, 2, 1) and you have 34 minutes.

ACTIVITY	TIME	EFFORT LEVEL
Interval 1	0:00–8:00	7–8
Recovery	8:00–10:00	5–6
Interval 2	10:00–17:00	7–8
Recovery	17:00–19:00	5–6
Interval 3	19:00–25:00	7–8
Recovery	25:00–27:00	5–6
Interval 4	27:00–32:00	7–8
Recovery	32:00–34:00	5–6
Interval 5	34:00–38:00	7–8
Recovery	38:00–40:00	5–6
Interval 6	40:00–43:00	7–8
Recovery	43:00–45:00	5–6
Interval 7	45:00–47:00	7–8
Recovery	47:00–49:00	5–6
Interval 8	49:00–50:00	7–8

More Ways to Play with Speed and Intensity

Swedish physiologists in the '60s were the first to cook up the idea that you can sprint faster and farther if you take breaks than if you go straight for the finish (well, duh). With that, intervals were born. But you don't need a stopwatch to do these workouts. You can also make up workouts based on how you feel, landmarks you see en route, or other time cues. The Swedish term for this type of made-up interval workout is *fartlek,* or "speed play." Here are some ideas to get you started.

Telephone Pole Pickups

Pick up the pace until you've passed a certain number of telephone poles (depending on how far apart they are and how long you want your intervals to be). Slow down for half as many poles, then repeat.

Punch Bug and Run

Just like the old backseat-of-the-car game, though these days you probably want to pick something slightly more common than a Volkswagen Beetle as your cue to throw in a surge. Pick something—a red car or a dog, for example—and every time you see one, speed up.

Be a Track Star

Head to the track at a high school and hit the starting line. Jog the curve, then run or walk as fast as you can down the straightaway. Continue this pattern. If you're biking, find a bike path with distances marked out along the way and pedal hard for half a mile, then slow down for the next half mile. (Of course these are just suggestions; you can make your intervals any distance you like.)

Did You Know? Stay Safe Headphones

You know that music can give your workout a boost, and research confirms it: Numerous studies have shown that listening to fast-paced music you love can make working out harder feel less, well, hard. Unfortunately, there are dangers to too much headphone wearing, especially during exercise. Blame it on trying to hear over our heavy breathing and pounding hearts, but even folks who listened at safe levels when sitting quietly cranked the volume to levels that made them more susceptible to hearing damage after just an hour and a half as soon as they hopped on a treadmill, say researchers from the University of Alberta in Canada. If you're exercising outdoors, headphones can also pose a safety issue if they prevent you from hearing what's going on around you. To protect yourself indoors and out, follow these guidelines.

For Indoor Workouts

Look for "noise isolating" headphones, which seal around your ear canal, muffling outside noise (like your gym's music and the treadmill's motor) so you can get pumped with less volume.

For Outdoor Workouts

Look for headphones in which the speaker sits up in front of or against the outside of your ear but doesn't go inside the ear canal.

Get Moved by Music

Make a playlist that alternates faster songs with slower ones (or just use whatever playlist pumps you up). Whenever a new song comes on, change speeds, picking it up for the duration of the song or slowing down until the next new song comes on. For shorter pickups, go fast just on the chorus.

Eating after 8 Weeks

If you have more weight to lose: Stick with the plan you've been following if you still have more pounds to lose. If you find you're feeling hungry, add another 200-calorie snack and make sure you're meeting your protein and fiber guidelines as well as drinking lots of water throughout the day.

If you're at your goal weight: Congratulations! The key now is to pinpoint the calorie level that will help you to stay at your current weight without regaining. For most women, that number will be around 1,600 to 1,800 calories a day, which you can do by adding one or two additional 200-calorie snacks per day from the program. Just remember, even if you've hit your goal, the diet guidelines you've been following to make sure you get enough protein to maintain muscle and enough fiber to feel full between meals will still help you to stay on track.

If you're not losing: Don't try to go below 1,400 calories per day because this plan centers around exercise, and cutting calories too much over time can decrease your metabolic rate and stall weight loss. Here are a few spots to troubleshoot to determine how you can get the scale headed in the right direction.

○ **Measure your portions.** Overestimating portion sizes (or forgetting to track bites here and there) could mean you're taking in more calories than you realize. Just an extra ¼ cup of rice or an extra ¼ tablespoon of almond butter a day is enough to stall weight loss in some people. Get both liquid and dry measuring cups and measuring spoons, and keep track of what you eat for a week (you don't have to do it forever, just long enough to identify any sneaky calories).

○ **Keep tabs on sodium.** Even though sodium doesn't cause fat gain, it can cause your weight to fluctuate considerably. While you don't want to drive yourself crazy with diet math, taking a few days to really read labels and add up the sodium you're consuming will help you to figure out where you might be blowing past the recommended 2,300 milligrams per day sodium limit suggested for this plan (as well as recommended by the American Dietetic Association).

○ **Be patient.** Don't expect instant results. The closer you are to your goal weight, the longer it may take for your body to jump into gear and drop the last few pounds. Patience is important in weight loss.

Conclusion

I hope you've enjoyed taking this journey with me to a fitter, stronger, lean-for-life body! With so many factors affecting our health that are beyond our control, simply picking up a pair of dumbbells and a rubber resistance band is truly one of the simplest ways to take control over both the way you look and feel now and the way your body ages over decades to come. For example, did you know that maintaining strong muscles—ideally starting now—is one of the best ways to steer clear of assisted living as you head into old age? And love 'em or hate 'em, doing your squats and lunges now helps to ensure you won't need a motorized lift chair down the line (after all, have you ever seen one that goes with your décor?). I hope these kinds of things are far from your mind, but they're just as important as—or more so than—the sexy sculpted arms, slimmed-down waistlines, and firmed-up backs our test panelists boasted about.

So now that you've completed this program, I have one more challenge for you. Whether you plan to continue this program or pick up another book and try something new, I want you to set a goal for yourself. Don't make it a goal that has anything to do with the scale. In fact, don't make it about what your body looks like at all. I want you to set a goal for what your body can *do*.

Maybe it's hiking to the top of a challenging trail near your house (or near a vacation spot your family is headed to in the coming year). Maybe it's finishing a 5-K without walking, or finishing a bike race in your best-ever time. You could even decide to ditch those 5-pound weights altogether by getting strong enough to use 8- or 10-pound weights and higher for all the exercises on this plan. Whatever you decide, this goal is all about you achieving something that makes you feel strong, more capable, and ready to conquer anything life throws your way. Good luck in your endeavors!

Appendix
Ⓐ

Eating for Energy 2-Week Sample Menu

After the Lighten-Up 7-Day Kickstart, you have a lot more flexibility in what you eat. As long as you follow the basic Eating for Energy guidelines in Chapter 8, no foods are off-limits. These 2 weeks of meals and snacks are designed to give you maximum energy and nutrition as your workout plans pick up steam. You can mix and match, add meals from the recipes in Chapter 8, or create your own meals to meet the guidelines. If you're feeling hungry on this diet, you can add a second snack. And don't forget to drink 2 glasses of water with each meal or snack to make sure you're well hydrated! Unless otherwise noted, meals and snacks in this menu serve one person.

Eating for Energy Week 1 Shopping List

If you've followed the 7-Day Lighten-Up Kickstart Menu exactly, you will have some nonperishable foods, such as olive oil and balsamic vinegar, left over. You may also have some of these foods in your pantry. So read through this list and check off what you already have on hand before heading to the store.

I've provided ounce measurements for some items because that's how they're sold in the stores. In a few cases, when you purchase the amount listed here, you will have a bit left over because of standard package sizing. Otherwise, this list provides the quantities of items you will need if you are following exactly the Eating for Energy Week 1 menu below. If you plan to make substitutions according to the guidelines we've given in Chapter 8, adjust your shopping list accordingly.

Produce

Romaine lettuce, one 10-ounce bag

Red onion, 2 tablespoons

Tomatoes, 2 medium

Grapes, 1 cup

Baby spinach, three 10-ounce bags

Garlic, 2½ cloves

Hass avocado, 1

Peach, 1 medium, or ½ cup unsweetened frozen slices

Strawberries, 3¼ cups (or 16 ounces) fresh or unsweetened frozen

Blueberries, ¾ cup (or 4.5 ounces) fresh or unsweetened frozen

Raspberries, 5¾ cups (or 20 ounces) fresh or unsweetened frozen

Tangerines or clementines, 3 medium

Green beans, 1 cup, fresh or plain frozen

Red potatoes, 2 large

Yellow or white onion, 1 small + 2 tablespoons

Carrots, baby, 2 cups

Kiwifruit, 2 medium

Red bell pepper, ¼ cup

Orange juice, ½ cup

Apple, green, 1 medium

Apples, red, 3 medium

Lemon juice, fresh or bottled, 2 tablespoons

Scallions, 2 medium

Silken tofu, light, 4 ounces

Dairy

Sour cream, reduced-fat, 2 ounces (or ¼ cup)

Greek yogurt, 0%, 14 ounces (or two 8-ounce cups)

Fat-free milk, 4¾ cups

Yogurt, plain, fat-free, 20 ounces (or 2½ cups)

Yogurt, flavored, light, 6 ounces (optional)

Cottage cheese, 1% or fat-free, no-salt-added, 6 ounces (or ¾ cup)

String cheese, light, two 1-ounce sticks

Eggs

Eggs, 8

Egg whites, 2 (or 2 ounces egg substitute)

Frozen Foods

Veggie burger, such as Boca Vegan Original, 1

Veggie sausage patty, such as Morningstar Farms (80 calories per patty), 4

Corn on the cob, medium, such as Green Giant Corn on the Cob Nibblers, 4 half ears

Bread/Cereal

Oats, ½ cup dry

Soft tortilla wrap, whole grain or whole wheat, 140 calories per wrap, 5

High-fiber cereal with at least 6 grams of fiber in 100 calories' worth (such as Kashi Good Friends or Barbara's Bakery Original), 1 cup

Bagel, whole wheat, 240 calories and at least 5 grams of fiber, 1

English muffin, whole wheat, 1

Roll, whole wheat, 100 or less calories and at least 4 grams of fiber per roll, 4

Dry Goods

Cooking spray

Canned salmon such as Chicken of the Sea brand Premium Skinless & Boneless Pink Salmon Pouch, 6 ounces (you can use cooked leftover salmon instead, if desired)

Olive oil, 3 tablespoons + 1 teaspoon

Canola oil, 1 tablespoon

Balsamic vinegar, 2 tablespoons

Red wine vinegar, 2 tablespoons

Dried currants, 5 tablespoons

Chickpeas or garbanzo beans, canned, no-salt-added, 2½ (15.5-ounce) cans (or 4½ cups)

Bread crumbs, plain dried, ¼ cup

Bread crumbs, seasoned dried, ½ cup

Almonds, whole, 3 tablespoons

Flaxseed, ground, 2 tablespoons (store in refrigerator)

Salsa, no-salt-added, 4 ounces

Tortilla chips, whole grain, about 140 calories' worth per 1-ounce serving, 2½ ounces (or 50 chips)

Peanut butter, 2 teaspoons

Black beans, canned, no-salt-added, two 15.5-ounce cans (or 3 cups)

Pineapple, diced, canned in juice or water, 16 ounces (or 2 cups)

Baked beans, canned, no-salt-added, 2½ (15.5-ounce) cans
(or 4 cups)

Barbecue sauce, 2 tablespoons

White vinegar, 1 tablespoon + 1 teaspoon

Sweet pickle relish, 1 tablespoon

Whole wheat flatbread-style cracker, about 45 calories each (such
as Wasa), 2

Honey, 3 tablespoons + 1 teaspoon (or 2½ ounces)

Walnuts, chopped, 3 tablespoons + 2 teaspoons (or 1 ounce)

Quinoa, dry, ¼ cup

Kidney beans, canned, no-salt-added, ½ cup (or 4½ ounces)

Mayonnaise, light, 2 tablespoons

Chunk light tuna, no-salt-added water pack, one 6-ounce can +
one 3-ounce can

Meal Replacement Bars

Organic Food Bar (Vegan, Original, or Active Greens flavor), 1 bar,
OR Clif bar (Chocolate Chip Peanut Crunch, Crunchy Peanut
Butter, or Peanut Toffee Buzz), 1

PowerBar Pria, any flavor, 1

Kashi GoLean Crunchy! Chocolate Caramel or Chocolate Peanut
bar, 1

Meat/Seafood

Chicken breasts, boneless skinless, raw, 1 pound

Flank steak, raw, 15 ounces

Roast beef, deli-sliced, reduced-sodium (such as Applegate Farms
Natural Roast Beef, or no more than 320 milligrams sodium per
2-ounce serving), 2 ounces

Pork tenderloin, raw, 1 pound

Turkey breast, deli-sliced (such as Applegate Farms brand, or no more than 360 milligrams sodium per 2-ounce serving), 2 ounces

Crab meat, raw, 12 ounces

Spices and Seasonings

Vanilla extract, ¾ teaspoon

Ground cinnamon, 1 teaspoon

Black pepper, about 2½ teaspoons

Cayenne pepper, ¼ teaspoon

Garlic powder, about ¾ teaspoon

Paprika, 1 teaspoon

Chili powder, 1½ teaspoons

Parsley, dried, ½ teaspoon

Dijon mustard, 4 teaspoons

Sage, dried, ⅛ teaspoon

Dill, dried, ½ teaspoon

Capers, ½ teaspoon

Ginger, ground, ½ teaspoon

Week 1 | Day 1

Breakfast: Denny's Scrambled Eggs and Pancakes

At Denny's, order the 4-ounce egg whites, scrambled, with an order of 2 wheat pancakes. Top them with one side order of grapes.

Breakaway Breakfast Option: Have 1 cup of sliced fruit or berries before your workout and skip the grapes at Denny's.

Per serving: 445 calories, 24 g protein, 94 g carbohydrates, 2 g total fat, 0 g saturated fat, 12 g fiber, 1,130 mg sodium

Lunch: Salmon Salad

Top 3 cups romaine lettuce with 1 medium tomato, diced; 2 tablespoons chopped red onion; 4 ounces cooked salmon, and ½ cup sliced grapes. Toss with 2 teaspoons olive oil and a splash of balsamic vinegar. Serve with 2 multigrain flatbread-style crackers.

Per serving: 388 calories, 28 g protein, 41 g carbohydrates, 14 g total fat, 3.5 g saturated fat, 9 g fiber, 750 mg sodium

Snack: Sweet Deviled Eggs (Serves 2)

Slice 6 hard-cooked eggs in half. Mash 2 of the yolks with 4 tablespoons light sour cream, ¼ teaspoon each vanilla extract and ground cinnamon, and 5 tablespoons dried currants or raisins. Refill egg halves with the mixture. Share 1 serving or save it for a snack later this week.

Per serving: 220 calories, 15 g protein, 20 g carbohydrates, 9 g total fat, 3.5 g saturated fat, 2 g fiber, 195 mg sodium

TIP: **Hate waste?** Leftover cooked egg yolks can be safely fed to your dog or cat (and will give their fur a nice shine to boot).

Dinner: Garbanzo Beans and Wilted Spinach (Serves 4)

Heat 1 tablespoon olive oil in a skillet over medium heat. Add 24 ounces fresh baby spinach and 2 cloves garlic, minced. Sauté for 3 to 4 minutes, or until spinach is wilted. Turn off heat. Add three 15-ounce cans (or 5¼ cups) no-salt-added chickpeas to spinach mixture along with ¼ cup plain bread crumbs, 1 teaspoon paprika, ½ teaspoon black pepper and 1 tablespoon balsamic vinegar. Turn heat to low, and heat until chickpeas are warmed through, 4 to 5 minutes.

Per serving: 408 calories, 20 g protein, 73 g carbohydrates, 6 g total fat, 0.5 g saturated fat, 20 g fiber, 340 mg sodium

Week 1 | Day 2

Breakfast: Hearty Oatmeal and Greek Yogurt

Top ¾ cup cooked oatmeal (½ cup dry + 1 cup of water) with ¼ teaspoon ground cinnamon, 2 tablespoons almonds, ¼ cup unsweetened frozen blueberries, thawed, and 2 tablespoons ground flaxseed. Serve with ¾ cup 0% Greek yogurt.

Breakaway Breakfast Option: Eat the Greek yogurt topped with the frozen blueberries.

Per serving: 413 calories, 26 g protein, 41 g carbohydrates, 18 g total fat, 2 g saturated fat, 10 g fiber, 75 mg sodium

Lunch: Veggie Burger with Chips and Salsa

Have a veggie burger topped with one-third of an avocado, chopped or mashed (save the rest for dinner), and 1 tablespoon no-salt-added salsa. On the side, have 2 cups romaine lettuce topped with a splash of balsamic vinegar and 1 teaspoon olive oil. Dip 20 whole grain tortilla chips (or 1 ounce) into another 3 tablespoons no-salt-added salsa.

Per serving: 407 calories, 20 g protein, 39 g carbohydrates, 23 g total fat, 4 g saturated fat, 13 g fiber, 582 mg sodium

Snack: Peach Smoothie

Combine 1⅓ cups fat-free milk with ½ cup unsweetened frozen or fresh peaches and 2 teaspoons peanut butter.

Per serving: 199 calories, 14 g protein, 26 g carbohydrates, 6 g total fat, 1.5 g saturated fat, 2 g fiber, 188 mg sodium

Dinner: Avocado and Black Bean Burrito (serves 4)

Slice the remaining ⅔ of the avocado from lunch and mix with 28 ounces (or 3 cups) canned no-salt-added black beans, rinsed and drained, and ½ teaspoon each ground cinnamon and chili powder. Divide mixture into 4 whole grain soft tortilla wraps. Serve with 2 cups pineapple (canned in juice or water or fresh).

Per serving: 394 calories, 16 g protein, 64 g carbohydrates, 8 g total fat, 1 g saturated fat, 15 g fiber, 198 mg sodium

Week 1 | Day 3

Breakfast: Veggie Wrap

Spread a whole grain soft tortilla wrap with 2 tablespoons fat-free plain yogurt mixed with ½ teaspoon each minced garlic clove and dried parsley. Fill wrap with ½ cup shredded romaine lettuce, 2 meatless sausage patties. Have 1 cup fresh or unsweetened frozen and thawed strawberries.

Breakaway Breakfast Option: Have half of the wrap.

Per serving: 399 calories, 27 g protein, 52 g carbohydrates, 9 g total fat, 1 g saturated fat, 10 g fiber, 710 mg sodium

Lunch: Energy Bar, Fruit and Milk

Have 1 Organic Food Bar or 1 Clif bar. Pair with ½ cup fresh or frozen and thawed unsweetened raspberries and 1 cup fat-free milk.

Per serving (depending on the bar you choose): 365–415 calories, 20–23 g protein, 53–61 g carbohydrates, 6 g total fat, 1–2.5 g saturated fat, 9–11 g fiber, 109–334 mg sodium

Snack: Tangerine and Grapes with Yogurt

Have 1 cup 0% Greek yogurt with 1 tangerine or clementine and ½ cup halved grapes.

Per serving: 197 calories, 21 g protein, 29 g carbohydrates, 0 g total fat, 0 g saturated fat, 2 g fiber, 88 mg sodium

Dinner: Chicken Breast and Baked Beans (Serves 4)

Coat a skillet with cooking spray and heat over low to medium heat. Season 1 pound raw chicken breast with black pepper and cook for 5 to 6 minutes on each side or until cooked through. Combine 3½ cups (or two 15-ounce cans), no-salt-added baked beans with 2 teaspoons Dijon mustard and 2 tablespoons barbecue sauce. Heat in the microwave on high for 1½ minutes, stir, and then continue heating for another 30 seconds. Serve with 2 cups steamed green beans.

Per serving: 387 calories, 36 g protein, 51 g carbohydrates, 4 g total fat, 1 g saturated fat, 13 g fiber, 244 mg sodium

Week 1 | Day 4

Breakfast: Cottage Cheese with Strawberries

Have ¾ cup no-salt-added fat-free or 1% cottage cheese with ¾ cup fresh or unsweetened frozen strawberries, thawed. Serve with ½ cup high-fiber cereal with 2 tablespoons pecans and ½ cup fat-free milk.

Breakaway Breakfast Option: Have the cereal and milk.

Per serving: 391 calories, 29 g protein, 49 g carbohydrates, 12 g total fat, 2 g saturated fat, 11 g fiber, 141 mg sodium

Lunch: Wendy's Salad and Baked Potato

Have the half-size Apple Pecan Chicken Salad topped with Italian Vinaigrette and half a plain baked potato. Use some of the Italian Vinaigrette on your baked potato if desired.

Note: If you mix and match meals, be sure to have this meal on a day where at least one meal or snack has no more than 2.5 g saturated fat and at least 9 g fiber.

Per serving: 385 calories, 22 g protein, 50 g carbohydrates, 18 g total fat, 4.5 g saturated fat, 7 g fiber, 803 mg sodium

Snack: Grab and Go Fruit and Cheese

Have 1 ounce light string cheese, 2 hard-boiled egg whites (feed the yolks to your cat or dog) and 2 tangerines or clementines.

Per serving: 194 calories, 17 g protein, 26 g carbohydrates, 4 g total fat, 2.5 g saturated fat, 3 g fiber, 356 mg sodium

Dinner: Spicy Beef Tenderloin, Potatoes, and Carrots (Serves 4)

On a plate, mix 1 teaspoon black pepper, ¼ teaspoon cayenne pepper, ½ teaspoon garlic powder and 1 teaspoon chili powder. Slice 15 ounces raw flank steak across the grain into long strips about 1/8-inch thick. Dredge each beef strip in the spice mixture. Coat a large skillet with cooking spray and heat over medium-high heat. Add steak, stirring for about 5 minutes or 2½ minutes on each side. Reduce heat to medium. Add 2 large red potatoes sliced in half; 1 small onion, chopped; ½ cup water, and 2 cups baby carrots. Cover and cook over medium heat for 20 minutes. Finish the meal with ½ cup fresh or unsweetened frozen raspberries, thawed, topped with 1 tablespoon plain fat-free yogurt per portion.

Per serving: 382 calories, 29 g protein, 46 g carbohydrates, 10 g total fat, 4 g saturated fat, 9 g fiber, 118 mg sodium

Week 1 | Day 5

Breakfast: Sausage Bagel

Have a whole wheat bagel filled with 1 meatless sausage patty and 2 slices tomato sprinkled with black pepper. Serve with 1 sliced kiwifruit.

Breakaway breakfast Option: Eat the kiwifruit alone.

Per serving: 394 calories, 22 g protein, 68 g carbohydrates, 5 g total fat, 1 g saturated fat, 14 g fiber, 711 mg sodium

Lunch: Roast Beef and Red Pepper Sandwich

Spread 1 toasted whole wheat English muffin with 2 tablespoons plain fat-free yogurt mixed with ⅛ teaspoon each dried sage and black pepper and 2 shakes of garlic powder. Fill with 2 ounces reduced-sodium lean sliced roast beef and ¼ cup thinly sliced red bell pepper. On the side have the rest of the bell pepper, sliced, and dip into ½ cup plain fat-free yogurt.

Per serving: 384 calories, 33 g protein, 48 g carbohydrates, 6 g total fat, 2 g saturated fat, 8 g fiber, 841 mg sodium

Snack: Savory Tuna Crackers

Mash 2½ ounces chunk light tuna packed in water, drained, with 1 teaspoon olive oil, a splash of white vinegar, and ½ teaspoon each dried dill and capers. Spread on or scoop with 2 multigrain flatbread-style crackers.

Per serving: 206 calories, 20 g protein, 20 g carbohydrates, 5 g total fat, 1 g saturated fat, 4 g fiber, 516 mg sodium

Dinner: Baked Pork Tenderloin and Apple Salad (Serves 4)

Preheat the oven to 350°F. Rub 1 pound pork tenderloin with ½ teaspoon ground ginger and bake for 30 minutes or until tender. While pork is baking, combine ½ cup orange juice, 1 tablespoon honey, and 1 teaspoon Dijon mustard. Remove pork from the oven, brush with orange juice mixture, and return to the oven to bake for another 10 minutes. Serve with 4 whole wheat rolls.

For the apple salad, finely chop 3 red apples and 1 green apple and toss with 3 tablespoons chopped walnuts and 2 tablespoons each red wine vinegar and honey.

Per serving: 399 calories, 31 g protein, 58 g carbohydrates, 7 g total fat, 1.5 g saturated fat, 9 g fiber, 229 mg sodium

Week 1 | Day 6

Breakfast: Quinoa and Berries

Make ¾ cup cooked quinoa (¼ cup dry). In a bowl, add quinoa, 1 cup fat-free milk, ½ cup each unsweetened frozen blueberries, thawed, and unsweetened frozen strawberries, thawed, and 2 teaspoons walnuts. On the side have 1 ounce light string cheese.

Breakaway Breakfast Option: Have half of the strawberries and half of the blueberries with the string cheese.

Per serving: 423 calories, 24 g protein, 63 g carbohydrates, 10 g total fat, 2.5 g saturated fat, 9 g fiber, 359 mg sodium

Speed-it-up tip: Leftover cooked quinoa can be frozen and reheated when needed. Just sprinkle with water and microwave.

Lunch: Southwest Spinach Salad

Combine 3 cups baby spinach, 2 ounces thinly sliced reduced-sodium turkey breast, and ½ cup no-salt-added kidney beans, drained. Toss with 3 tablespoons no-salt-added salsa and 1 tablespoon olive oil, and break 10 whole grain tortilla chips (or ½ ounce) over top.

Per serving: 399 calories, 27 g protein, 38 g carbohydrates, 18 g total fat, 2.5 g saturated fat, 15 g fiber, 517 mg sodium

Snack: Energy Bar and Yogurt

Have 1 cup 0% Greek yogurt with ¼ cup fresh or unsweetened frozen raspberries stirred in, and 1 PowerBar Pria, any flavor.

Per serving: 206 calories, 18 g protein, 26 g carbohydrates, 4 g total fat, 2–2.5 g saturated fat, 3 g fiber, 140 mg sodium

Dinner: Fast Crispy Crab Cakes (Serves 4)

Combine ¾ pound raw blue crab meat with 1 teaspoon Dijon mustard, ½ cup seasoned bread crumbs, 2 tablespoons lemon juice, 4 egg whites, 2 scallions, chopped (use both the white and green parts), and 2 tablespoons light mayonnaise. Form mixture into 4 large patties or 8 small patties. In a skillet, heat 1 tablespoon canola oil and sauté crab cakes over medium heat on each side until cooked through, about 4 to 5 minutes on each side. Serve with 4 half ears corn on the cob and 4 cups fresh or unsweetened, frozen raspberries, thawed.

Per serving: 432 calories, 27 g protein, 59 g carbohydrates, 10 g total fat, 1.5 g saturated fat, 12 g fiber, 660 mg sodium

Week 1 | Day 7

Breakfast: Bar and Yogurt

Have 1 Kashi GoLean Crunchy! Chocolate Caramel or Chocolate Peanut bar. Pair with 1 cup 0% Greek plain yogurt mixed with 1 cup fresh or unsweetened frozen strawberries, thawed, and topped with 1 tablespoon almonds.

Breakaway Breakfast Option: Eat just the bar.

Per serving: 436 calories, 24 g protein, 78 g carbohydrates, 6 g total fat, 5 g saturated fat, 9 g fiber, 416 mg sodium

Lunch: Tangy Tuna and Tortillas

Mix 6 ounces chunk light tuna packed in water, drained, with 1 tablespoon each sweet pickle relish and white vinegar and 2 tablespoons chopped onion. Scoop tuna with 20 whole grain tortilla chips (or 1 ounce). Have ¾ cup fresh or unsweetened frozen raspberries, thawed.

Per serving: 415 calories, 48 g protein, 36 g carbohydrates, 9 g total fat, 1.5 g saturated fat, 9 g fiber, 312 mg sodium

Snack: Kiwifruit and Silky Tofu Smoothie

Blend 4 ounces light silken tofu, undrained; 1 sliced kiwifruit; 1 cup fat-free milk; 1 teaspoon honey; and ½ teaspoon vanilla extract.

Per serving: 200 calories, 17 g protein, 31 g carbohydrates, 1 g total fat, 0.5 g saturated fat, 2 g fiber, 218 mg sodium

Dinner: Applebee's Grilled Chicken Caesar Salad

Have the half-size Grilled Chicken Salad with dressing on the side. Get the Bleu Cheese, Dijon Honey Mustard, Mexi-Ranch, or Buttermilk Ranch and use half. Order a side of Fresh Fruit and the Kid's Steamed Broccoli.

Per serving (depending on the dressing you choose): 370–415 calories, 28 g protein, 39–46 g carbohydrates, 12–18 g total fat, 3–4 g saturated fat, 9 g fiber, 580–695 mg sodium

Eating for Energy Week 2 Shopping List

Again, this list provides the quantities of items you will need if you are following exactly the Eating for Energy Week 2 menu below. You may have many nonperishables left over from the previous week. If you plan to make substitutions according to the guidelines we've given in Chapter 8, adjust your shopping list accordingly.

Produce

Orange juice, ¼ cup

Pear, 1 large

Grapes, 1 cup

Strawberries, fresh or unsweetened frozen, 3 ounces (or ½ cup)

Romaine lettuce, 12 cups (or two 10-ounce bags)

Red bell pepper, 1 large

Mixed berries, fresh or unsweetened frozen, 9 ounces (or 1½ cups)

Raspberries, fresh or unsweetened frozen, 2½ ounces (or ½ cup)

Blueberries, fresh or unsweetened frozen, 5 ounces (or 1 cup)

Tomatoes, 3 medium

Garlic, ½ teaspoon

Banana, 1 small

Mixed baby greens, 4 ounces (or 3 cups)

Tangerine or clementine, 1

Kiwifruit, 2

Baby spinach, three 12-ounce bags (or 13 cups)

Potatoes, Idaho or Yukon Gold, 4 medium

Radishes, 6 medium

Arugula, 6 cups

Chives, chopped, ⅓ cup (or 0.5 ounce)

Green onion or scallions, ½ cup (or 2 ounces)

Broccoli, 2 cups (or 7 ounces)

Orange or yellow bell pepper, 1 large

Edamame, fresh or frozen without shell, 3 cups (or 16 ounces)

Dairy

Fat-free milk, 2⅔ cups

Light Muenster cheese, ¾ ounce

Cheddar cheese, 2% fat, slices, 1 ounce

Cheddar cheese, reduced-fat, shredded, ½ ounce

Ricotta cheese, fat-free, ⅔ cup

Yogurt, plain, fat-free, 2½ cups (or 22 ounces)

String cheese, light, one 1-ounce stick

Parmesan cheese, grated, or asiago cheese, grated, 3 tablespoons + 1 teaspoon (or one small container)

Cottage cheese, 1% or fat-free, no-salt-added, 6 ounces (or ¾ cup)

Greek yogurt, 0%, 1 cup

Mozzarella cheese, reduced-fat, shredded, 4 ounces (or 1 cup)

Cream cheese, reduced-fat, 1 tablespoon

Refrigerator Case

Whole wheat cheese tortellini with at least 6 grams fiber per 1-cup serving (such as Buitoni Whole Wheat Three Cheese), 15 ounces (or 4 cups)

Eggs

4 eggs

5 egg whites (or ⅔ cup or 5 ounces egg substitute)

Frozen Foods

Whole grain waffles, 90 calories and at least 1.5 grams fiber each (such as Van's), 2

Healthy Choice Café Steamers Balsamic Garlic Chicken, Healthy Choice Café Steamers Grilled Basil Chicken, or Healthy Choice Café Steamers Lemon Garlic Chicken and Shrimp **OR** Lean Cuisine

Market Creations Chicken Poblano (or select any frozen entrée with 700 or less milligrams sodium, 285 calories, 16 grams or more protein, 5.5 grams fiber, and 3 or less grams saturated fat)

Veggie sausage patty, 80 calories (such as Morningstar Farms), 1

Lima beans, 23 ounces (or 4 cups)

Breads/Cereal

High-fiber cereal, 6 or more grams fiber in 100 calories' worth (such as Kashi Good Friends or Barbara's Bakery Original), ¾ cup

Whole wheat bread, 80 calories and 3 grams fiber per slice (such as Martin's Whole Wheat Potato Bread or Weight Watchers 100% Whole Wheat Bread), 6 slices

Kellogg's Special K Protein Plus **OR** Kashi GoLean Protein and High Fiber Cereal, 2¼ cups

Whole wheat pita, 4", 1

Whole wheat English muffin, 1

Whole wheat bagel, 240 calories and 5 or more grams fiber (such as Thomas' Whole Wheat Bagels), 1

Dry Goods

Cooking spray, 3 spritzes

Olive oil, 7 tablespoons + 1 teaspoon

Canola oil, 1 tablespoon

Sesame oil, 1½ tablespoons

Balsamic vinegar, 2 tablespoons

Whole wheat flatbread-style cracker, 45 calories (such as Wasa), 4

Minestrone soup, no-salt-added (such as Health Valley), 2 cups (or 16 ounces)

Cannellini beans, canned, no-salt-added, two 15.5-ounce cans + ½ cup (or 3 cups)

Black beans, canned, no-salt-added, 5 ounces (or ½ cup)

Kidney beans, canned, no-salt-added, 4½ ounces (or ½ cup)

Garbanzo beans, canned, no-salt-added, 11 ounces (or 1¼ cups)

Red wine vinegar, ½ cup

Honey, 2 teaspoons

Ground coffee, caffeinated or decaffeinated, 1 heaping tablespoon

Soy milk, light, vanilla, 2 cups

Peanut butter, 1 teaspoon

Almonds, slivered, 3 tablespoons

Pecans, 5 tablespoons

Mixed nuts, 2 tablespoons

Canned salmon (such as Chicken of the Sea brand Premium Skinless & Boneless Pink Salmon Pouch), 2 ounces (use cooked leftover salmon instead, if desired)

Dried currants or raisins, 3 tablespoons

Lentil soup, no-salt-added canned (such as Health Valley brand), 50 ounces (or 6 cups)

Applesauce, unsweetened, 6 ounces (or ¾ cup)

Cranberries, dried, 2 tablespoons

Pineapple, diced, canned in juice or water, 6 ounces (or ¾ cup)

Artichokes, jarred, 2 cups

Spaghetti sauce, no-salt-added, 9 ounces (or 1 cup)

Brown rice, 1 cup dry (6.75 ounces)

Soy sauce, reduced-sodium, lite, 2 tablespoons

Meal Replacement Bars

Organic Food Bar (Vegan, Original, or Active Greens flavor) **OR** Clif bar (Chocolate Chip Peanut Crunch, Crunchy Peanut Butter, or Peanut Toffee Buzz)

Meat/Seafood

Ham, deli-sliced, reduced-sodium, 480 or less milligrams sodium per 2 ounces (such as Applegate Farms brand), 11 ounces

Roast beef, deli-sliced, reduced-sodium, 320 or less milligrams sodium per 2 ounces (such as Applegate Farms brand), 2 ounces

Turkey, deli-sliced, reduced-sodium, 360 or less milligrams sodium (such as Applegate Farms), 2 ounces

Spices/Seasonings

Vanilla extract, ¾ teaspoon

Dill, dried, ½ teaspoon

Capers, 1 tablespoon + 1 teaspoon

Ground cinnamon, ¼ teaspoon

Ground nutmeg, ¼ teaspoon

Chocolate syrup, 1 tablespoon (such as Hershey's brand)

Oregano, dried, 2¼ teaspoons

Basil, dried, ¾ teaspoon

Rosemary, dried, 2 teaspoons

Black pepper, 1½ teaspoons

Week 2 | Day 8

Breakfast: Cheesy French Toast (Serves 2)

Whisk 2 eggs and 2 egg whites with ¼ teaspoon each cinnamon and nutmeg, ½ teaspoon vanilla extract,and ½ cup fat-free milk. Heat a skillet over low to medium heat with 1 tablespoon canola oil. Dip 4 slices whole wheat bread into egg mixture and cook on each side until egg is set. Have 1½ slices with 1 large pear, chopped, and ¾ ounce light Muenster cheese over top or on the side. (Share or save the rest; if saving, keep the egg mixture in the refrigerator for 1 day and reheat in the microwave for 45 seconds on high or in the oven at 250°F for 4 to 5 minutes.)

Breakaway Breakfast Option: Eat the pear.

Per serving: 409 calories, 22 g protein, 45 g carbohydrates, 16 g total fat, 4 g saturated fat, 8 g fiber, 480 mg sodium

Lunch: Minestrone Soup and Crackers

Serve 2 cups no-salt-added minestrone soup with 2 multigrain flatbread-style crackers, 1 ounce 2% Cheddar cheese, and ½ cup grapes.

Per serving: 413 calories, 20 g protein, 67 g carbohydrates, 10 g total fat, 4.5 g saturated fat, 11 g fiber, 504 mg sodium

Snack: Chocolate Strawberry Shake

Blend together 1⅔ cups fat-free milk with ½ cup unsweetened frozen strawberries, ¼ teaspoon vanilla extract, and 1 tablespoon chocolate syrup.

Per serving: 222 calories, 14 g protein, 40 g carbohydrate, 1 g total fat, 0.5 g saturated fat, 2 g fiber, 187 mg sodium

Dinner: Hearty Antipasto Salad (Serves 4)

Combine 12 cups romaine lettuce; 3 cups (or 1¼ 15-ounce cans) no-salt-added cannellini beans, rinsed and drained; 9 ounces reduced-sodium ham, thinly sliced into strips; 1 cup thinly sliced red bell pepper; and 1 tablespoon plus 1 teaspoon capers. Toss with 4 tablespoons each olive oil and red wine vinegar and 2 teaspoons each dried oregano and dried rosemary.

Per serving: 380 calories, 21 g protein, 33 g carbohydrates, 19 g total fat, 3.5 g saturated fat, 10 g fiber, 528 mg sodium

Week 2 | Day 9

Breakfast: Waffles and Honey Berry Ricotta

Toast 2 frozen whole grain waffles and spread with ⅔ cup fat-free ricotta cheese mixed with 1 teaspoon honey. Top with 1 cup fresh or unsweetened frozen and thawed mixed berries.

Breakaway Breakfast Option: Have 1 waffle with 2 tablespoons ricotta cheese and honey mixture and ½ cup berries.

Per serving: 381 calories, 25 g protein, 62 g carbohydrates, 8 g total fat, 0.5 g saturated fat, 10 g fiber, 534 mg sodium

Lunch: Bar, Fruit, and Yogurt

Have 1 Organic Food Bar or 1 Clif bar. Pair with ½ cup fresh or frozen unsweetened and thawed raspberries mixed with ⅔ cup fat-free plain yogurt.

Per serving (depending on the bar you choose): 374–424 calories, 21–24 g protein, 53–61 g carbohydrates, 8 g total fat, 1–2.5 g saturated fat, 9–11 g fiber, 133–358 mg sodium

Snack: Vanilla Soy Latte

Combine 1 cup brewed coffee with 2 cups warmed light vanilla soy milk. Serve with 1 multigrain flatbread-style cracker, spread with 1 teaspoon peanut butter.

Per serving: 199 calories, 16 g protein, 21 g carbohydrates, 7 g total fat, 1 g saturated fat, 2 g fiber, 329 mg sodium

Dinner: Quick Chicken Dinner

Select one of the frozen entrées mentioned in the grocery list and prepare. Preheat the oven to 250°F, place 3 tablespoons slivered almonds on a piece of foil, and bake for 3 to 4 minutes or until they turn light brown. Sprinkle the almonds on your entrée or serve on the side.

Per serving (depending on the frozen entrée): 366–416 calories, 20–44 g protein, 38–44 g carbohydrates, 15–17 g total fat, 2–3 g saturated fat, 8–10 g fiber, 540–640 mg sodium

Week 2 | Day 10

Breakfast: Blueberry-Pecan Cereal and Milk

Have 1 cup of Special K Protein Plus (or 130 calories' worth of another high-protein cereal) with ½ cup fat-free milk, 1 cup fresh or unsweetened frozen and thawed blueberries, and 2 tablespoons pecans. On the side, have 1 ounce light string cheese.

Breakaway Breakfast Option: Have ½ cup of the blueberries and 1 ounce light string cheese.

Per serving: 410 calories, 28 g protein, 49 g carbohydrates, 17 g total fat, 3 g saturated fat, 11 g fiber, 440 mg sodium

Lunch: Quick Three-Bean Stew

Combine ½ cup each no-salt-added canned cannellini beans, black beans, and kidney beans. Rinse and drain all beans and toss with 2 teaspoons olive oil; a splash of balsamic vinegar; 1 medium tomato, chopped; and ¼ teaspoon each dried oregano and dried basil. Warm in the microwave on high for 1½ minutes, stirring once.

Per serving: 416 calories, 21 g protein, 60 g carbohydrates, 11 g total fat, 1.5 g saturated fat, 20 g fiber, 441 mg sodium

Snack: Mini Salmon Pizza

Preheat the oven to 350°F. Drizzle 1 teaspoon olive oil over a small (4" diameter) whole wheat pita, sprinkle with 2 ounces salmon, ½ teaspoon minced garlic, ½ teaspoon dried dill, and 2 teaspoons grated asiago or Parmesan cheese. Heat for 3 to 4 minutes or until crust is browned.

Per serving: 203 calories, 14 g protein, 17 g carbohydrates, 9 g total fat, 3 g saturated fat, 2 g fiber, 480 mg sodium

Dinner: Chicken Fajitas

Order the Chicken Fajitas at Chili's. Have the chicken, all of the veggies, and the black beans. Do not eat the sour cream, cheese, guacamole, rice, and flour tortillas.

Per serving: 430 calories, 48 g protein, 42 g carbohydrates, 10 g total fat, 2 g saturated fat, 13 g fiber, 1,870 mg sodium

Week 2 | Day 11

Breakfast: Egg Muffin

Toast 1 whole wheat English muffin. Fill with 3 egg whites scrambled in ½ teaspoon olive oil and 1 veggie sausage patty. Serve with 1 small banana and ½ cup grapes.

Breakaway Breakfast Option: Have the banana.

Per serving: 403 calories, 28 g protein, 62 g carbohydrates, 7 g total fat, 1.5 g saturated fat, 9 g fiber, 843 mg sodium

Lunch: Dried Fruit, Nuts, and Mixed Baby Greens Salad

Top 3 cups mixed baby greens with ¾ cup fat-free or 1% no-salt-added cottage cheese, 2 tablespoons dried currants or raisins, 2 tablespoons mixed nuts, and 1 tangerine or clementine, sectioned. Drizzle with ½ teaspoon olive oil and balsamic vinegar.

Per serving: 387 calories, 28 g protein, 44 g carbohydrates, 14 g total fat, 3 g saturated fat, 8 g fiber, 69 mg sodium

Snack: Roast Beef and Cheese Cracker

Top 1 multigrain flatbread-style cracker with 2 ounces lean deli roast beef and ½ ounce 2% Cheddar cheese. Serve with 1 sliced kiwifruit.

Per serving: 198 calories, 18 g protein, 17 g carbohydrates, 6 g total fat, 3 g saturated fat, 4 g fiber, 403 mg sodium

Dinner: Lentil Soup and Baked Potato (Serves 4)

Preheat the oven to 375°F. Have 6 cups (or 3½ 14.5-ounce cans) no-salt-added canned lentil soup. Mix in 1 cup baby spinach and top with 2 tablespoons plus 2 teaspoons grated Parmesan cheese before heating. Pierce 4 medium brown potatoes several times with a fork and place on a piece of foil. Bake for 1 hour or until slightly soft and golden brown. Season each potato with black pepper and 3 tablespoons plain, fat-free yogurt mixed with 1 teaspoon dried chives.

Per serving: 297 calories, 17 g protein, 59 g carbohydrates, 4 g total fat, 1 g saturated fat, 14 g fiber, 134 mg sodium

Week 2 | Day 12

Breakfast: IHOP Omelet

Order the Simple & Fit Veggie Omelet with Fresh Fruit.

Breakaway Breakfast option: Eat 1 cup of sliced fruit or berries and skip the fruit side at IHOP.

Per serving: 320 calories, 21 g protein, 40 g carbohydrates, 10 g total fat, 1 g saturated fat, 8 g fiber, 420 mg sodium

Lunch: Grilled Turkey, Cheddar, and Tomato with Cranberry Applesauce

Coat a skillet with cooking spray and heat over low to medium heat. Spray outsides of 2 slices of whole wheat bread with cooking spray, fill with 2 ounces low-sodium sliced turkey, ½ ounce shredded reduced-fat Cheddar cheese, and 2 slices tomato and place in pan. Cook on each side for about 3 to 4 minutes or until bread is lightly browned and cheese melts. Serve with ¾ cup unsweetened applesauce mixed with 2 tablespoons dried cranberries.

Note: If you prefer to take this sandwich to work and eat it cold, skip the cooking step and use sliced cheese (it will stay together better without melting).

Per serving: 393 calories, 33 g protein, 63 g carbohydrates, 7 g total fat, 3 g saturated fat, 11 g fiber, 831 mg sodium

Snack: Tropical Yogurt

Have 1 cup 0% Greek yogurt with ¾ cup pineapple chunks canned in juice or water, drained.

Per serving: 201 calories, 21 g protein, 30 g carbohydrates, 0 g total fat, 0 g saturated fat, 2 g fiber, 86 mg sodium

Dinner: Marinated Artichoke and Radish Salad with Mozzarella (Serves 4)

Whisk together ⅓ cup red wine vinegar with 2 tablespoons olive oil and 1 teaspoon black pepper. Combine 4 cups cooked from frozen or fresh lima beans; 2 cups jarred artichokes, drained and cut in half; 6 fresh radishes, sliced; 6 cups fresh arugula; ¼ cup fresh chives, chopped; and ¾ cup shredded reduced-fat mozzarella cheese. Toss with the vinegar dressing.

Tip: Make this dish in the morning to give the marinade plenty of time to flavor this salad. Toss before serving. In a pinch, the salad can be made just before serving.

Per serving: 391 calories, 21 g protein, 53 g carbohydrates, 11 g total fat, 3 g saturated fat, 18 g fiber, 693 mg sodium

Week 2 | Day 13

Breakfast: Pecan Cereal

Serve ¾ cup high-fiber cereal with 1¼ cups plain or flavored light fat-free yogurt and 3 tablespoons pecans.

Breakaway Breakfast Option: Have ¾ cup of the yogurt with 1 tablespoon pecans.

Per serving: 381 calories, 20 g protein, 48 g carbohydrates, 14 g total fat, 1.5 g saturated fat, 10 g fiber, 296 mg sodium

Lunch: Au Bon Pain Salad

Have the Mandarin Sesame Chicken Salad. Skip the dressing and use a splash of vinegar, if desired. Pair it with 1 slice of Whole Wheat Multigrain Bread.

Per serving: 440 calories, 26 g protein, 58 g carbohydrates, 11 g total fat, 2 g saturated fat, 9 g fiber, 755 mg sodium

Snack: Berry Smoothie

Blend ½ cup unsweetened frozen mixed berries with 1 cup 0% Greek plain yogurt, 1 teaspoon honey, and ¼ cup orange juice.

Per serving: 204 calories, 21 g protein, 32 g carbohydrates, 0 g total fat, 0 g saturated fat, 2 g fiber, 87 mg sodium

Dinner: Cheese Tortellini (Serves 4)

Prepare 4 cups whole wheat cheese tortellini. Top with 1 cup no-salt-added spaghetti sauce and ¼ cup reduced-fat shredded mozzarella cheese and divide between 4 plates. Serve each portion with a side of 3 cups baby spinach topped with balsamic vinegar.

Per serving: 401 calories, 20 g protein, 52 g carbohydrates, 12 g total fat, 4.5 g saturated fat, 10 g fiber, 587 mg sodium

Week 2 | Day 14

Breakfast: Savory Ham Bagel

Spread a whole wheat bagel with 1 tablespoon low-fat cream cheese. Sprinkle with ½ teaspoon dried or 1 teaspoon fresh chives, and fill with 2 ounces reduced-sodium ham. Serve with 1 sliced kiwifruit.

Breakaway Breakfast Option: Have half of the bagel sandwich.

Per serving: 397 calories, 22 g protein, 65 g carbohydrates, 7 g total fat, 3 g saturated fat, 12 g fiber, 848 mg sodium

Lunch: Easy Garbanzo Beans and Tomato

Combine 1¼ cups (or 10.5 ounces) no-salt-added canned garbanzo beans (rinsed and drained) with 1 medium tomato, chopped; ½ teaspoon dried basil; 1 teaspoon olive oil; and 1 tablespoon balsamic vinegar.

Per serving: 402 calories, 19 g protein, 65 g carbohydrates, 7 g total fat, 1 g saturated fat, 14 g fiber, 85 mg sodium

Snack: Cereal and Dried Fruit

Have high-protein cereal with 1 tablespoon dried currants or raisins.

Per serving (depending on which cereal you choose): 209 calories, 15–17 g protein, 44 g carbohydrates, 1 g total fat, 0 g saturated fat, 7–13 g fiber, 107 mg sodium

Dinner: Fried Rice with Veggies and Edamame (Serves 4)

Coat a skillet with cooking spray and heat over medium heat. Add 2 eggs and stir until lightly scrambled. Remove from skillet. In the same skillet, heat 1½ tablespoons sesame oil, turn down the heat to low to medium, and add ½ cup chopped green onion (use green and white part of the onion), 2 cups broccoli florets, 1 cup chopped orange or yellow bell pepper, and 3 cups edamame without the pod, fresh or frozen. Sauté, stirring often, until vegetables are softened, about 7 to 10 minutes. Add 3 cups cooked brown rice to the pan and 2 tablespoons lite reduced-sodium soy sauce and stir until rice is warmed through. Add eggs and heat for another minute or two.

Per serving: 425 calories, 20 g protein, 54 g carbohydrates, 14 g total fat, 2 g saturated fat, 11 g fiber, 399 mg sodium

Appendix

B

Tone Every Inch Logs

Keeping track of your strength and cardio workouts as well as what you eat can help you stay accountable (it's harder to sneak an extra cupcake when you know you have to write it down, and to skip a workout when you know there will be a record!). It also makes it easier to follow (and celebrate!) your progress when you can look back and see how much more weight you're able to lift or how much faster and farther you can go in your cardio workouts compared with the beginning of the program. You can see samples of each of these logs at the end of Chapters 3, 4, 5, and 8, but here are blank forms for you to photocopy and use.

Band Workout Log

Week of program: ◯ **Date:** _____

EXERCISE	REPS	WEIGHT USED (COLOR OF BAND)	OBSERVATIONS/ CHALLENGES
Two-Way Row			
Pickup and Shrug			
Chest Press			
Side Leg-Lift Crunch			
Cheerleader Press			
Skater Side Twist			
Pullover and Crunch			
Lunge Repeater			
Butt Kicker			
Squat and Curl			

Triple-Duty Toning Workout Log

Week of program: ⬭ **Date:** _____

EXERCISE	REPS	WEIGHT USED (COLOR OF BAND AND/OR SIZE OF DUMBBELL)	OBSERVATIONS/ CHALLENGES
Triple-Duty Two-Way Row			
Triple-Duty Pickup and Shrug			
Triple-Duty Chest Press			
Triple-Duty Side Leg-Lift Crunch			
Triple-Duty Cheerleader Press			
Triple-Duty Skater Side Twist			
Triple-Duty Pullover and Crunch			
Triple-Duty Lunge Repeater			
Triple-Duty Butt Kicker			
Triple-Duty Squat and Curl			

Weekly Exercise Overview

Week of program: ◯   **Date:** _____

DAY	WORKOUTS	TIME OF DAY	DURATION	OBSERVATIONS/ CHALLENGES	DAILY TOTAL EXERCISE TIME

Daily Food Log

Week of program: ◯   **Date:** _____

MEAL	FOOD/ BEVERAGE CONSUMED	CALORIES/ PROTEIN/ FIBER	TIME OF DAY	OBSERVATIONS/ CHALLENGES
Breakfast				
Lunch				
Snack				
Dinner				
Optional Extra Snack				

Acknowledgments

This book would never have come to be without the help of the many wonderful people around me.

Thanks to my intrepid team of exercise science students at Ithaca College: Matt Baluzy, Kristen Demers, Hanna Foley, Alana Koehler, John Silver, and last but certainly not least, Sarah Simunovich, who led the charge. Thanks to Miranda Kaye, PhD, for giving me access to a great crew of students, and to Gary Sforzo, PhD, for agreeing to oversee this project.

Thanks to my amazing editors, Andrea Au Levitt, Katie Wyszynski, and Marielle Messing for reining in my ramblings when needed, always asking great questions, and, along with designer Carol Angstadt, shaping a manuscript 20 times longer than the magazine stories I'm used to writing into this great-looking book before you.

To Michele Stanten, the former fitness director of *Prevention* magazine, for showing me the book-writing ropes before this project was even on the horizon, and for always having both great expectations and great faith in my abilities as a writer.

To all the many researchers, exercise physiologists, trainers, and physicians I've called and e-mailed over the years, especially my personal guru of strength-training research Wayne Westcott, PhD; thank you for patiently helping this English major make sense of the science of sculpting (and cardio, and so many other things).

To my now-stronger-than-ever team of test panelists—Colleen Barnes, Jen Brown, Merry Buckley, Mary Dennis, Sherri Dunham, Madeline Estill, Ethna Hinrichsen, Donna Holzbaur, Lisa McCutcheon, Barbara Terrell, Katrina Walker, and Ann Warde—thanks for taking the leap with me. I couldn't be more proud of what you've all accomplished.

And finally, to my husband, Sam: Thanks for your unmatched skill at knowing just how to talk me down from a cliff when I was buried in seemingly impossible deadlines, for your unflagging support when even I had my doubts, and for your good sense to realize that when you're about to embark on writing a book, it's the perfect time to adopt a puppy. Thanks for being on my team; I couldn't have done it without you.

Index

Boldface page references indicate photographs. Underscored references indicate boxed text.

D